AF449283

CAMPTOTHECINS: NEW ANTICANCER AGENTS

Edited by

Milan Potmesil, M.D., Ph.D.
New York University School of Medicine
New York, New York

and

Herbert Pinedo, M.D.
Department of Oncology
Free University
Amsterdam, The Netherlands

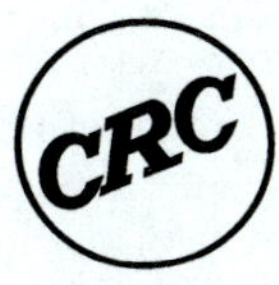

CRC Press
Boca Raton Ann Arbor London Tokyo

Library of Congress Cataloging-in-Publication Data

Catalog record is available from the Library of Congress

© 1995 by CRC Press, Inc.

No claim to original U.S. Government works
International Standard Book Number 0-8493-4764-5
Printed in the United States of America 1 2 3 4 5 6 7 8 9 0
Printed on acid-free paper

CONTRIBUTORS

Daniel Abigerges, M.D.
Department of Adult Medicine
Institut Gustave-Roussy
Villejuif, France

Toshiwo Andoh, M.D.
Laboratory of Biochemistry
Aichi Cancer Center
Nagoya, Japan

Jean-Pierre Armand, M.D.
Department of Adult Medicine
Institut Gustave-Roussy
Villejuif, France

Jos Beijnen, M.D.
Department of Pharmacy
Slotervaart Hospital and Netherlands
  Cancer Institute
Amsterdam, The Netherlands

Marie-Christine Bissery, Ph.D.
Rhône-Poulenc Rorer
Vitry-Sur-Seine, France

Maureen de Boer-Dennert, M.D.
Department of Medical Oncology
Rotterdam Cancer Institute
Rotterdam, The Netherlands

Wim ten Bokkel Huinink, M.D.
Department of Medical Oncology
Antoni van Leeuwenhoek
Amsterdam, The Netherlands

Roland Bugat, M.D.
Centre Claudius-Régaud
Toulouse, France

Howard A. Burris, III, M.D.
Cancer Therapy and Research Center
San Antonio, Texas
 and
Brooke Army Medical Center
Oncology Clinic
Fort Sam Houston, Texas

Guy G. Chabot, Ph.D.
Clinical Pharmacology Laboratory
U 140 INSERM and URA 147 CNRS
Villejuif France

Michel Clavel, M.D.
Centre Léon-Bérard
Lyon, France

Stephane Culine, M.D.
Hôpital Saint-Louis
Paris, France

Ross C. Donehower, M.D.
Johns Hopkins Cancer Center
Baltimore, Maryland

Jean-Marc Extra, M.D.
Hôpital Saint-Louis
Paris, France

Kim M. Fehir, Ph.D.
The Stehlin Foundation for Cancer
  Research
St. Joseph Hospital
Houston, Texas

Suzanne M. Fields, Pharm.D.
Cancer Therapy and Research Center
San Antonio, Texas

Marcel de Forni, M.D.
Department of Adult Medicine
Institut Gustave-Roussy
Villejuif, France

Beppino C. Giovanella, Ph.D.
The Stehlin Foundation for Cancer
  Research
St. Joseph Hospital
Houston, Texas

Alain Gouyette, Ph.D.
Clinical Pharmacology Laboratory
U 140 INSERM and URA 147 CNRS
Villejuif, France

Heine Hansen, M.D.
Department of Oncology
Rigshospitalet
Copenhagen, Denmark

Nicholas J. Harris, B.S.
The Stehlin Foundation for Cancer
  Research
St. Joseph Hospital
Houston, Texas

Patrice Hérait, M.D.
Laboratoire Roger Bellon
Neuilly-Sur-Seine, France

Hellmuth R. Hinz, Ph.D.
The Stehlin Foundation for Cancer
  Research
St. Joseph Hospital
Houston, Texas

Howard S. Hochster, M.D.
Department of Medicine
New York University School of
  Medicine
New York, New York

Peter de Ipolyi, M.D.
The Stehlin Foundation for
  Cancer
St. Joseph Hospital
Houston, Texas

Ineke Koier, M.D.
EORTC New Drug Development
  Office
Amsterdam, The Netherlands

Anthony J. Kozielski, B.S.
The Stehlin Foundation for Cancer
  Research
St. Joseph Hospital
Houston, Texas

Irwin H. Krakoff, M.D.
Division of Medicine
M.D. Anderson Cancer Center
Houston, Texas

John G. Kuhn, Pharm.D.
Department of Pharmacology
The University of Texas Health Sciences
  Center
San Antonio, Texas

Leroy F. Liu, M.D.
Department of Pharmacology
Robert Wood Johnson Medical
  School
Piscataway, New Jersey

Aurelico Lorico, M.D.
Comprehensive Cancer Center
Yale University School of Medicine
New Haven, Connecticut

Birthe Lund, M.D.
Department of Oncology
Rigshospitalet
Copenhagen, Denmark

Alice K. Marcee, B.S.
The Stehlin Foundation for Cancer
  Research
St. Joseph Hospital
Houston, Texas

Michel Marty, M.D.
Hôpital Saint-Louis
Paris, France

Anne Mathieu-Boué, M.D.
Laboratoire Roger Bellon
Neuilly-Sur-Seine, France

Franco Muggia, M.D.
Norins Cancer Center
University of Southern California
Los Angeles, California

Ethan A. Natelson, M.D.
The Stehlin Foundation for Cancer
  Research
St. Joseph Hospital
Houston, Texas

Kosuke Okada, M.D.
Department of Blood Transfusion
Hiroshima University Hospital
Hiroshima, Japan

Herbert M. Pinedo, M.D.
Department of Medical Oncology
Free University Hospital
Amsterdam, The Netherlands

Andre Planting, M.D.
Department of Medical Oncology
Rotterdam Cancer Institute
Rotterdam, The Netherlands

Yves Pommier, M.D.,Ph.D.
Laboratory of Molecular
  Pharmacology
National Cancer Institute
National Institutes of Health
Bethesda, Maryland

Milan Potmesil, M.D., Ph.D.
Department of Radiology
New York University Medical Center
New York, New York

Hilde Rosing, M.D.
Department of Pharmacy
Slotervaart Hospital and Netherlands
  Cancer Institute
Amsterdam, The Netherlands

Mace L. Rothenberg, M.D.
Division of Oncology
Department of Medicine and Oncology
University of Texas Health Sciences
  Center
  and
Cancer Therapy and Research
  Center
San Antonio, Texas

Eric K. Rowinsky, M.D.
Department of Pharmacology
Johns Hopkins Oncology Center
Baltimore, Maryland

Armado Ruiz-Razura
The Stehlin Foundation for Cancer
  Research
Houston, Texas

John S. Stehlin, M.D.
The Stehlin Foundation for Cancer
  Research
St. Joseph Hospital
Houston, Texas

Tetsuo Taguchi, M.D.
Emeritus Professor
Osaka University
Osaka, Japan

Akihiko Tanizawa, M.D.
Department of Pediatrics
Fukui Medical College
Fukui, Japan

Thomas P. Trezona, M.D.
The Stehlin Foundation for Cancer
  Research
Houston, Texas

Dana Vardeman
The Stehlin Foundation for Cancer
  Research
Houston, Texas

Jaap Verweij, M.D.
Department of Medical Oncology
Rotterdam Cancer Institute
Rotterdam, The Netherlands

Daniel D. Von Hoff, M.D.
Department of Medicine
Division of Oncology
University of Texas
Health Sciences Center
  and
Cancer Therapy and Research Center
San Antonio, Texas

Monroe E. Wall, Ph.D.
Research Triangle Institute
Research Triangle Park, North Carolina

Mansukh C. Wani, Ph.D.
Research Triangle Institute
Research Triangle Park, North Carolina

CONTENTS

INTRODUCTION

There are numerous defense mechanisms in the biological world, used by fungi, bacteria, and plants to protect themselves against their adversaries. The production of toxins, such as the alkaloids isolated from *Camptotheca acuminata* of the *Nyssaceae* family, may be part of such complex systems which have been in place throughout evolution.

Over the past several years, a new class of anticancer agents has been identified and developed. The camptothecins, synthetic and semisynthetic derivatives of a plant alkaloid, inhibit a cellular enzyme DNA topoisomerase I and trigger a cascade of events leading to apoptosis and programmed cell death. Currently, several drugs of this class are in various stages of preclinical and clinical testing: the parent compound 20(S)-camptothecin (CAM, NSC 94600) and the analogs 9-amino-20(S)-camptothecin (9-AC, NSC 603071), CPT-11 (irinotecan) and topotecan (NSC 609699) (Table 1). Additional derivatives are still being tested in the laboratory. This surge of activity, which is opening a promising field of cancer chemotherapy, was preceded by discoveries in biology and biochemistry of DNA topoisomerases as well as by considerable progress in drug synthesis.

The rallying point for this book was the Fourth Conference on DNA Topoisomerases in Therapy, held in New York City in October 1992. The presentations concerning camptothecins have been developed into book chapters. Most of the chapters were prepared by teams developing and testing the camptothecins in the United States, Japan, and Europe.

CAM and methoxylated or carboxylated forms of this alkaloid are found in the wood, bark, and fruit of *Camptotheca acuminata*.[1] (Table 1). An effusion, injectable, or powder prepared from the tree have been used in traditional Chinese medicine in treatment of various illnesses including tumors.[2] Among thousands of plants analyzed during the 1960s in a search for steroids suitable for the synthesis of cortisone, CAM and naturally occurring analogs were discovered and analyzed by Monroe Wall, Mansukh Wani and colleagues.[1,3] CAM and analogs were also found in several other plant families.[4-7] In 1958, an extract from the Camptotheca tree was tested by the National Cancer Institute and its antitumor activity established in experimental systems.[8] Subsequent studies by Susan Horwitz, David Kessel and other researchers showed the inhibition of both DNA and RNA synthesis by CAM, and this was accompanied in cultured mammalian cells by a reversible fragmentation of DNA.[9-15] Upon drug removal, the inhibition of high molecular weight RNA synthesis was reversed totally, whereas DNA synthesis was restored only partially.[10,11] This led to a suggestion that CAM cytotoxic effects are cell-cycle specific, directed at the S-phase.[14] In preparation for clinical testing, CAM, a compound with limited water solubility, was formulated as a water-soluble CAM-Na$^+$ (NSC-100880). Clinical studies complemented by drug pharmacology were initiated in the late 1960s, and results of Phase I and partial II trials published in 1970–1972.[16-19] Although antitumor activity was observed among patients with gastrointestinal cancer in some trials, reported bone marrow and nonhematological toxicities were judged severe enough to preclude further testing. At that time, laboratory research of the CAM molecule[20] confirmed an earlier observation[8] which established the importance of the lactone E-ring for drug cytotoxicity and the inactivity of the open-ring carboxylated CAM-Na$^+$ in media with neutral pH. Further application of this essential observation to preclinical and clinical research had to wait another twenty years.

In the late 1980s, several developments renewed the interest in camptothecins: an enzyme, DNA topoisomerase I, was identified as a cellular target of CAM[21,22] and analogs;[23,24] a structure-activity relationship was determined for semisynthetic and totally synthetic CAM derivatives;[23,24] an overexpressed topoisomerase I was found in advanced stages of human colon adenocarcinoma[25] and other malignancies[26] but not in normal

Table 1   20(S)-Camptothecin (a) hydrolyzed form (B), and analogs

(a)

(b)

Drug	Form	MW	C7	C9	C10	C11
CAM, 20(S)-camptothecin	(a)	348	H	H	H	H
CAM-Na+, camptothecin sodium salt	(b)	388	H	H	H	H
9-AC, 9-amino-20(S)-camptothecin	(a)	363	H	NH_2	H	H
CPT-11, 7-ethyl-10-[4-(1-piperidino)-1-piperidino]carbonyloxy-camptothecin	(a)	585	C_2H_5	H	O-C=O (piperidino-piperidino)	H
Topotecan, 9-dimethylamino-methyl-10-hydroxycampto-thecin	(a)	421	H	$(CH_3)_2NHCH_2$	OH	H

tissues; and semisynthetic and totally synthetic analogs 9-AC (NSC 603071)[27] and 10,11-MDC[28] have shown an unprecedented effectiveness against human colon adenocarcinoma carried by immunodeficient nude mice.[25,29,30] At that time, CPT-11 and topotecan were prepared and tested in experimental settings.[31,32] In the early 1990s, both latter drugs were introduced into clinical trials.[33,34] 9-AC was developed in collaboration between a research group and the National Cancer Institute, and Phase I clinical trials initiated in early 1993. In addition, there is a Phase I trial of CAM given orally.

During the past twenty-five years, various aspects of topoisomerase I biochemistry, molecular biology, genetics, and topo I-CAM interaction have been studied. Some of the observations came in place during recently initiated efforts to develop camptothecins as anticancer agents effective against refractory cancers. Research of camptothecins represents an active field, with promising results seen in patients with inherently resistant malignancies such as non-small cell lung or colon cancers. Research of camptothecins exemplifies drug development which, within a few years, progressed from a laboratory curiosity to clinical application. The following listing of book chapters is accompanied by brief synopsis:

Table 2 Chronology of preclinical and clinical development of CAM (based on published full articles or book chapters)

		Ref.
1966	Active agent 20(S)-camptothecin isolated and its structure established.	1
1966–1970	Extracts from *Camptotheca acuminata* have antitumor activity	1, 3
1970–1972	Phase I/II clinical trials of camptothecin sodium salt.	16–19
1985–1988	20(S)-Camptothecin inhibits DNA topoisomerase I.	21, 22
1986–1991	Analogs 9-aminocamptothecin, CPT-11, and topotecan synthesized and tested.	27, 30–32
1988–1989	DNA topoisomerase I is elevated in several types of human malignancies.	25, 26
1989	The enzyme is inhibited by biologically active analogs.	23, 24
1989–1993	Unprecedented effectiveness of 9-aminocamptothecin, 20(S)-camptothecin, and other analogs against human cancer in xenografts.	25, 29, 30
1991–1993	Analogs and 20(S)-camptothecin are in clinical trials.	33, 34

Chapter 1 — Biochemistry of Camptothecin, by *Leroy F. Liu.* Following an overview of DNA topoisomerase I biochemistry, biology, and genetics, the chapter discusses the intricacies of camptothecin-topoisomerase I interaction, a mechanism of enzyme inhibition, cell killing, and drug resistance.

Chapter 2 — Camptothecin and Analogs: From Discovery to Clinic, by *Monroe E. Wall and Mansukh C. Wani,* provides detailed historical background of the camptothecin discovery and describes synthesis and testing of camptothecin analogs with ring-A substituents, their water-soluble derivatives, and other new structural types.

Chapter 3 — Twenty Years Later: Review of Clinical Trials with Camptothecin Sodium (NSC-100880), by *Franco Muggia.* Camptothecin sodium salt, a water-soluble congener, was briefly tested in Phase I and II trials. The results of these trials, conducted in the early 1970s, are analyzed in retrospect. Although early tumor-specific effects were reported, the general consensus based on detected toxicities led to the discontinuation of clinical testing. Several considerations of camptothecin scheduling and pharmacology are also presented.

Chapter 4 — Preclinical Development of 20(S)-camptothecin, 9-aminocampto-thecin, and Other Analogs, by *Milan Potmesil and Beppino C. Giovanella.* The drugs have shown an unprecedented effectiveness against a variety of xenografts of resistant human cancers, against liver or central nervous system metastases, and against tumor cells with expressed MDR1 phenotype. Studies indicate that the plasma level of its lactone, sustained above a threshold for a prolonged time, is necessary for optimal therapeutic effects. Currently, Phase I trials of 9-aminocamptothecin have been initiated.

Chapter 5 — Phase I Clinical Trial and Pharmacokinetic Results with Oral Administration of 20(S)-camptothecin, by *John S. Stehlin et al.* Unlike camptothecin sodium salt, the lactone form delivered via gastrointestinal tract has shown excellent effectiveness against a spectrum of human cancer xenografts. Currently, a Phase I study of oral camptothecin lactone was initiated, and data on bioavailability, toxicities, and objective responses were provided.

Chapter 6 — Clinical Studies of CPT-11 in Japan, by *Tetsuo Taguchi.* Phase II clinical trials of CPT-11 in Japan have established the effectiveness against a variety of resistant malignancies. The most impressive are the results obtained in patients with

4

non-small cell lung cancer and with advanced gynecological or colorectal cancer. Dose-limiting toxicities are also discussed.

Chapter 7 — Clinical Trials and Pharmacokinetics of CPT-11 in the United States, by *Mace L. Rothenberg et al.* The drug has been tested in a Phase I study on two different schedules, a 90-min infusion every two or three weeks. Dose-limiting toxicities included diarrhea and other gastrointestinal symptoms. CPT-11 and its biologically active metabolite SN-38 have relatively long terminal half-lives in plasma, and this is an advantage for the treatment with S-phase specific drugs. In order to confirm a wide spectrum of activities reported, CPT-11 entered Phase II evaluation against a variety of refractory solid tumors and leukemia as well as combination studies, with, e.g., 5-fluorouracil or cisplatin.

Chapter 8 — Clinical Trials and Pharmacology Studies of CPT-11 and Its Active Metabolite SN-38 in France: Preliminary Pharmacokinetic-Pharmacodynamic Relationship, by *Guy G. Chabot et al.* Phase I trials evaluated a 90-min and 5-d continuous infusion of the drug. CPT-11 has a triphasic elimination pattern with a terminal half-life of 16–18 h, which may ensure desirable sustained plasma levels of the active metabolite. The pharmacokinetics can be valuable for the prediction of gastrointestinal and hematological toxicities.

Chapter 9 — Topotecan Clinical Trials in the United States, by *Howard Hochster.* The National Cancer Institute-sponsored research of topotecan included Phase I evaluation of over forty different protocols and schedules. The drug is entering Phase II studies in patients with non-small lung cancer and refractory cancer of the ovary, and Phase I trials of the combination with taxol, another effective natural product with anticancer properties, etoposide, or cisplatin were also initiated.

Chapter 10 — Clinical Trials of Topotecan in Europe, by *Jaap Verweij et al.* Data are available on initial Phase I trials using 24-h continuous infusion every three weeks, or daily injections for 5 consecutive days repeated every three weeks. Leukopenia was dose-limiting, while thrombocytopenia occurred less frequently. The latter protocol is currently applied in Phase II studies to patients with small-cell lung or metastatic colorectal cancer.

Chapter 11 — Camptothecins: Dose-Limiting Toxicities and Their Management, by *Howard A. Burris, III et al.* Granulocytopenia is a dose-limiting toxicity of topotecan, while the primary toxicity limiting dose escalation of CPT-11 is the development of diarrhea and/or granulocytopenia. A considerable effort has been made to establish the etiology of diarrhea induced by CPT-11 and to prevent or control it by supportive care regimens. Application of biological stimulators of hematopoieses is planned for Phase II trials of topotecan, while an effective control of gastrointestinal toxic symptoms will be applied in Phase II testing of CPT-11.

Chapter 12 — Cellular Determinants of Sensitivity and Resistance to Camptothecins, by *Yves Pommier et al.* A discussion of factors involved in cell sensitivity or resistance to camptothecins is followed by an overview of resistant cell lines developed *in vitro*. The review includes data on two camptothecin-resistant lines, CPT-K5 and DC3F/C-10, with structural changes of the gene which encodes DNA topoisomerase I. The chapter includes a discussion of possible implications of the findings for molecular biology of camptothecins.

Chapter 13 — The Perspectives, by the Editors. A discussion of presented observations and future trends: combination treatments for specific types of resistant cancers, a strategy for overcoming the resistance to camptothecins, and the dose intensification of treatments, and the development of a second generation of camptothecins.

REFERENCES

1. **Wall, M. E., Wani, M. C., Cook, C. E., Palmer, K. H., McPhail, A. T., and Sim, G. A.,** Plant antitumor agents. I. The isolation and structure of camptothecin, a novel alkaloidal leukemia and tumor inhibitor from *Camptotheca acuminata, J. Amer. Chem. Soc.,* 88, 3888, 1966.

2. **Huang, S.-Y., Ed.,** *Seven Hundred Herbal Prescriptions for Cancer Medicine Treatment* (in Chinese), Bada Educational and Cultural Publishers, Taipei, Chinese Rep., 1986.

3. **Perdue, R. E., Jr., Smith, R. L., Wall, M. E., Hartwell, J. L., and Abbott, B. J.,** *Camptotheca acuminata* Decaisne *(Nyssaceae),* source of camptothecin, an antileukemic alkaloid, Technical Bulletin, No. 1415, U.S. Department of Agriculture, Agricultural Research Service, Washington, D.C., 1970.

4. **Govindachari, T. R. and Viswanathan, N.,** 9-Methoxycamptothecin. A new alkaloid from *Mappia foetida* miers, *Ind. J. Chem.,* 10, 453, 1972.

5. **Govindachari, T. R. and Viswanathan, N.,** Alkaloids of *Mappia foetida, Phytochemistry,* 11, 3529, 1972.

6. **Arisawa, M., Gunasekera, S. P., Cordell, G. A., and Farnsworth, N. R.,** Plant anticancer agents XXI. Constituents of merrilliodendron megacarpum, *Planta Med.,* 43, 404, 1981.

7. **Gunasekera, S. P., Badawi, M. M., Cordell, G. A., Farnsworth, N. R., and Chitnis, M.,** Potential anticancer agents. X. Isolation of camptothecin and 9-methoxy-camptothecin from *Ervatamia heyneana, J. Nat. Prod.,* 42, 475, 1979.

8. **Wall, M. E.,** Alkaloids with antitumor activity, in *International Symposium on Biochemistry and Physiology of the Alkaloids,* Mothes, K., Schreiber, K., and Schutte, H. R., Eds., Academie-Verlag, Berlin, 1969, 77.

9. **Bosmann, H. B.,** Camptothecin inhibits macromolecular synthesis in mammalian cells but not in isolated mitochondria of *E. coli, Biochem. Biophys. Res. Commun.,* 41, 1412, 1970.

10. **Horwitz, S. B., Chang, C.-K., and Grollman, A. P.,** Studies on camptothecin. 1. Effects on nucleic acid and protein synthesis, *Mol. Pharmacol.,* 7, 632, 1971.

11. **Kessel, D.,** Effects of camptothecin on RNA synthesis in leukemia L1210 cells, *Biochem. Biophys. Acta.,* 246, 225, 1971.

12. **Wu, R. S., Kumar, A., and Warner, J. R.,** Ribosomal formation is blocked by camptothecin, a reversible inhibitor of RNA synthesis, *Proc. Natl. Acad. Sci. U.S.A.,* 68, 3009, 1971.

13. **Abelson, H. T. and Penman, S.,** Selective interruption of high molecular weight RNA synthesis in HeLa cells by camptothecin, *Natl. New Biol.,* 237, 144, 1972.

14. **Kessel, D., Bosmann, H. B., and Lohr, K.,** Camptothecin effects on DNA synthesis on murine leukemia cells, *Biochim. Biophys. Acta.,* 269, 210, 1972.

15. **Horwitz, M. S. and Horwitz, S. B.,** Intracellular degradation of HeLa and adenovirus type 2 DNA induced by camptothecin, *Biochem. Biophys. Res. Commun.,* 45, 723, 1971.

16. **Gottlieb, J. A., Guarino, A. M., Call, J. B., Oliverio, V. T., and Block, J. B.,** Preliminary pharmacologic and clinical evaluation of camptothecin sodium (NSC-100880), *Cancer Chemother. Rep.,* 54, 461, 1970.

17. **Muggia, F. M., Creaven, P. J., Hansen, H. H., Cohen, M. H., and Sealwry, O. S.,** Phase I clinical trial of weekly and daily treatment with camptothecin (NSC-100880): correlation with preclinical studies, *Cancer Chemother. Rep.,* 56, 515, 1972.

18. **Moertel, C. G., Schutt, A. J., Reitemeier, R. J., and Hahn, R. G.,** Phase II study of camptothecin (NSC-100880) in the treatment of advanced gastrointestinal cancer, *Cancer Chemother. Rep.,* 56, 95, 1972.

19. **Gottlieb, J. A. and Luce, J. K.,** Treatment of malignant melanoma with camptothecin (NSC-100880), *Cancer Chemother. Rep.,* 56, 103, 1972.

20. **Danishefsky, S., Quick, J., and Horwitz, S. B.,** Synthesis and biological activity in the camptothecin series, *Tetrahedron Letters,* 27, 2525, 1973.

21. **Hsiang, Y.-H., Hertzberg, R., Hecht, S., and Liu, L. F.,** Camptothecin induces protein-linked DNA breaks via mammalian DNA topoisomerase I, *J. Biol. Chem.,* 260, 14873, 1985.

22. **Hsiang, Y.-H. and Liu, L. F.,** Identification of mammalian topoisomerase I as an intracellular target of the anticancer drug camptothecin, *Cancer Res.,* 48, 1722, 1988.

23. **Jaxel, C., Kohn, K. W., Wani, M. C., Wall, M. E., and Pommier, Y.,** Structure-activity study of the actions of camptothecin derivatives on mammalian topoisomerase I. Evidence for a specific receptor site and for a relation to antitumor activity, *Cancer Res.,* 49, 1465, 1989.

24. **Hsiang, Y.-H., Liu, L. F., Wall, M. E., Wani, M. C., Kirshenbaum, S., Silber, R., and Potmesil, M.,** DNA topoisomerase I-mediated DNA cleavage and cytotoxicity of camptothecin analogs, *Cancer Res.,* 49, 4385, 1989.

25. **Giovanella, B. C., Stehlin, J. S., Wall, M. E., Wani, M. C., Nicholas, A. W., Liu, L. F., Silber, R., and Potmesil, M.,** DNA topoisomerase I-targeted chemotherapy of human colon cancer in xenografts, *Science,* 246, 1046, 1989.

26. **Potmesil, M., Hsiang, Y.-H., Liu, L. F., Bank, B., Grossberg, H., Kirschenbaum, S., Forlenzar, T. J., Penziner, A., Kanganis, D., Knowles, D., Traganos, F., and Silber, R.,** Resistance of human leukemic and normal lymphocytes to drug-induced DNA cleavage and low levels of DNA topoisomerase II, *Cancer Res.,* 48, 3537, 1988.

27. **Wall, M. E., Wani, M. C., Natschke, S. M., and Nicholas, A. W.,** Plant antitumor agents. 22. Isolation of 11-hydroxycamptothecin from *Camptotheca acuminata* Decne: total synthesis and biological activity, *J. Med. Chem.,* 29, 1553, 1986.

28. **Wani, M. C., Nicholas, A. W., Manikumar, G., and Wall, M. E.,** Plant antitumor agents. 25. Total synthesis and anti-leukemic activity of ring A substituted camptothecin analogs. Structure-activity correlations, *J. Med. Chem.,* 30, 1774, 1987.

29. **Potmesil, M., Giovanella, B. C., Liu, L. F., Wall, M. E., Silber, R., Stehlin, J. S., Jr., Hsiang, Y.-H., and Wani, M. C.,** Preclinical studies of DNA topoisomerase I-targeted 9-amino and 10, 11-methylenedioxy camptothecins, in *DNA Topoisomerases in Cancer,* Potmesil, M. and Kohn, K. W., Eds., Oxford University Press, New York, 1991, 299.

30. **Potmesil, M., Giovanella, B. C., Wall, M. E., Liu, L. F., Silber, R., Stehlin, J. S., Wani, M. C., and Hochster, H.,** Preclinical development of DNA topoisomerase I inhibitors in the United States, in *Molecular Biology of DNA Topoisomerases and its Application to Chemotherapy,* Andoh, T., Ikeda, H., and Oguro, M., Eds., CRC Press, Nagoya, Japan, 1993, chap. 29.

31. **Kunimoto, T., Nitta, K., Tanaka, T., Uehara, N., Baba, H., Takeuchi, M., Yokokura, T., Sawada, S., Miyasaka, T., and Mutai, M.,** Antitumor activity of 7-ethyl-10-[14-(1-piperidino)-1-piperidino] carbonyloxy-camptothecin, a novel water-soluble derivative of camptothecin, against murine tumors, *Cancer Res.,* 47, 5944, 1987.

32. **Kingsbury, W. D., Boehm, J. C., Jakas, D. R., Holden, K. G., Hecht, S. M., Gallagher, G., Caranfa, M. J., McCabe, F. L., Faucette, L. F., Johnson, R. K., and Hertzberg, R. P.,** Synthesis of water-soluble (aminoalkyl) camptothecin analogs: inhibition of topoisomerase I and antitumor activity, *J. Med. Chem.,* 34, 98, 1991.

33. **Negoro, S., Fukuoka, M., Masuda, N., Takada, M., Kusunoki, Y., Matsui, K., Takifuji, N., Kudoh, S., Niitani, H., and Taguchi, T.,** Phase I study of weekly intravenous infusions of CPT-11, a new derivative of camptothecin, in the treatment of advanced non-small cell lung cancer, *J. Natl. Cancer Inst.,* 83, 1164, 1991.

34. **Rowinsky, E., Grochow, L., Hendricks, C., Sartorius, S., Ettinger, D., McGuire, W., Forastiere, A., Hurowitz, L., Easter, V., and Donehower, R.,** Phase I and pharmacologic study of topotecan (SK&F 104864): a novel topoisomerase I inhibitor, *Proc. Amer. Soc. Clin. Oncol.,* 10, 93, 1991.

Chapter 1

Biochemistry of Camptothecin

Leroy F. Liu

CONTENTS

I. INTRODUCTION

Camptothecin and some of its analogs appear to be promising anticancer drugs with a new mode of action. The molecular target for camptothecin has been identified to be DNA topoisomerase I, an important nuclear enzyme for various DNA functions including transcription and replication. Several key steps involved in the action of camptothecin have also been partially elucidated. At the target level, camptothecin specifically inhibits the breakage/rejoining reaction of DNA topoisomerase I. The inhibition appears to be specific for the rejoining step, which leads to the accumulation of the putative covalent reaction intermediate, a reversible topoisomerase I-camptothecin-DNA ternary complex (the cleavable complex). At the cell level, the interaction between DNA replication forks, and the ternary complex triggers cell death and many other cellular responses. In addition to S-phase specific cell killing, camptothecin can also induce cell differentiation and transcription of certain growth- and differentation-related genes. It is possible that this may contribute to the antitumor activity of camptothecin. Another unique feature of camptothecin is its broad antitumor spectrum against many solid tumors. This has been attributed to the ability of camptothecin to overcome MDR1-mediated resistance completely. While the exact antitumor mechanism of camptothecin remains to be determined, the identification of topoisomerase I as an important molecular target for cancer therapeutics has facilitated the understanding of the antitumor activity of camptothecin and is likely to stimulate the development of new topoisomerase I-targeting drugs in the future.

II. EARLY RESEARCH ON CAMPTOTHECIN

The impressive activity of camptothecin has led to intensive investigation into its mode of action in the early 1970s. Campotothecin was shown to inhibit both DNA and RNA synthesis.[1-3] While inhibition of DNA synthesis appears irreversible or partially reversible, inhibition of RNA synthesis is highly reversible.[2,3] Another striking effect of camptothecin is its rapid fragmentation of chromosomal DNA.[4] Interestingly, fragmentation of chromosomal DNA is highly reversible upon drug removal.[4] At the cell level, camptothecin kills S-phase cells specifically and induces extensive sister chromatid exchanges and chromosomal abberations.[5,6] All these cellular effects of camptothecin remained unexplained until the identification of topoisomerase I as the molecular target of camptothecin.[7,8]

The antiviral activity of camptothecin has also been demonstrated. Camptothecin inhibits replication of both SV40 virus and adenovirus.[4,9] However, *vaccinia* viral DNA replication is unaffected by camptothecin. It has since been determined that due to its cytoplasmic life cycle, *vaccinia* virus encodes its own topoisomerase I which is camptothecin-resistant.[10] Interestingly, a single base mutation in the *vaccinia* topoisomerase I gene can convert the camptothecin-resistant *vaccinia* enzyme into a camptothecin-sensitive topoisomerase.[11]

Total synthesis of camptothecin has been achieved, and many derivatives of camptothecin have also been made.[12-15] Among them, derivatives with substitutions at the A-ring positions often exhibited higher activity. Modifications of the E-ring often lead to inactivation. Some of the promising camptothecin derivatives are shown in Figure 1.

III.   THE MOLECULAR TARGET OF CAMPTOTHECIN: TOPOISOMERASE I

Two fundamentally different types of topoisomerases have been identified and characterized from both prokaryotic and eukaryoptic cells.[16-18] Type I DNA topoisomerases (see Table 1) are enzymes which catalyze the topoisomerization reactions (e.g., relaxation/supercoiling, knotting/unknotting, and catenation/decatenation) of DNA via transient enzyme-linked, single-strand breaks. They characteristically change the DNA linking number in steps of one. Type II DNA topoisomerases (see Table 1) are enzymes which catalyze the topoisomerization reactions (e.g., relaxation/supercoiling, knotting/unknotting, and catenation/decatenation) of DNA via transient enzyme-linked, double-strand breaks. They characteristically change the linking number of DNA in steps of two. So far, three mammalian DNA topoisomerases (TOP1, TOP2α, and TOP2β) have been identified and characterized.[19-21]

In 1984, the molecular target for a number of intercalative (e.g., adriamycin, m-AMSA, and ellipticine) and non-intercalative (VP-16 and VM-26) antitumor drugs have been identified to be DNA topoisomerase IIα, a 170 kDa (M_r) nuclear enzymes which are essential for DNA replication and RNA transcription.[22,23] These antitumor drugs characteristically induce protein-linked DNA breaks in cultured mammalian cells. In addition, these protein-linked DNA breaks disappear rapidly upon removal of drugs from treated cells.[22,23] The similarity between topoisomerase II drugs and camptothecin in their unusual effect on chromosomal DNA fragmentation has initially led to the testing of camptothecin as a topoisomerase II drug.[7] Surprisingly, camptothecin had no effect on topoisomerase II. More extensive analysis has led to the identification of topoisomerase I as the nuclear target of camptothecin.[7,24]

Mammalian DNA topoisomerase I is a monomeric protein of 100 kDa, and its gene has been isolated and mapped to chromosome 20q12-13.2.[25-28] Topoisomerase I is a type I DNA topoisomerase and catalyses relaxation of both positively and negatively supercoiled DNA with about equal efficiency. The relaxation reaction does not require any energy cofactor and can occur in the presence of EDTA. Its primary function is probably to remove excessive supercoils generated during DNA processes such as replication and transcription.[29,30] The preferential association of topoisomerase I with transcribed regions of genes also support an intimate role of topoisomerase I in transcription.[31] More recently, topoisomerase I has been shown to interact directly with TBP (TATA-binding protein).[32] The human DNA topoisomerase I cDNA (see Figure 2) encodes a polypeptide of 765 amino acids.[27] The N-terminal one-third of topoisomerase I is highly charged (about 60% charged amino acids) and is nonessential for the catalytic activity.[27] The active site tyrosine has been located to amino acid residue #723 of the human enzyme.[33]

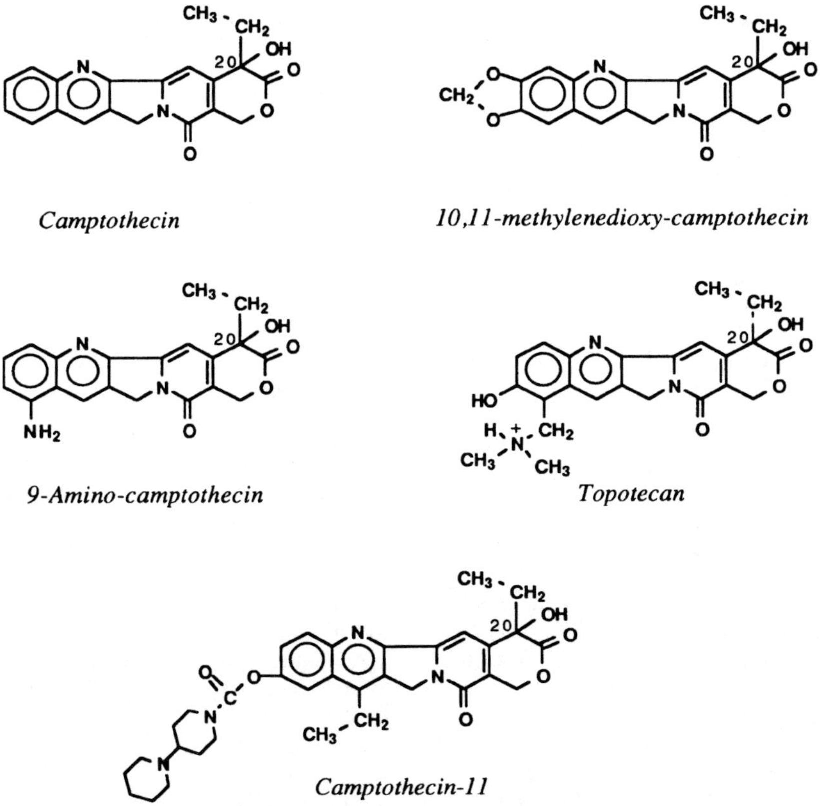

Camptothecin

10,11-methylenedioxy-camptothecin

9-Amino-camptothecin

Topotecan

Camptothecin-11

Figure 1 Chemical structures of some camptothecins.

High levels of topoisomerase I have been detected in all nucleated eukaryotic cells. While the overall protein level of topoisomerase I does not change very significantly during different phases of the cell cycle, the mRNA level of topoisomerase I appears to increase more dramatically as cells enter proliferation or are stimulated with the tumor promoter PMA. Like c-myc and several other protooncogenes, super-induction of topoisomerase I mRNA is also observed upon simultaneous inhibition of protein synthesis.[34,35] It is interesting that higher levels of topoisomerase I have been detected in surgical specimens of colon tumors as compared to normal mucosa of colon.[36]

IV. MECHANISM OF INHIBITION

The topoisomerase I relaxation reaction can be conceptually divided into two steps (see Figure 3). This reaction is initiated by a nucleophilic attack on the phosphate of the phosphodiester linkage by the tyrosine hydroxyl (#723 of the human DNA topoisomerase I), resulting in an enzyme-linked single-strand break in which the enzyme is covalently linked to the 3′-phosphoryl end of the broken DNA strand.[37] In this stage, the phosphodiester linkage opposite to the transient break can presumably swivel (the extent of this swiveling is not known but may be limited by the presence of the covalently bound topoisomerase I). Following swiveling or "strand passing", the rejoining reaction is initiated by a nucleophilic attack on the tyrosyl phosphate by the 5' hydroxyl to release the tyrosine

Table 1 Major DNA topoisomerases from prokaryotes and eukaryotes

Enzymes (Type)	Gene	Organism	Hallmark Reaction	Structure
Topo I (I)	*topA*	eubacteria	relaxation of (–) supercoils	monomer
Topo III (I)	*topB* (or *top3*)	eubacteria (or yeast)	relaxation of (–) supercoils	monomer
Reverse gyrase (I)		archebacteria	positive supercoiling	monomer
Topo V (I)		archebacteria	relaxation of (+,–) supercoils	monomer
Topo I (I)	*top1*	eukaryotes	relaxation of (+,–) supercoils	monomer
Gyrase (II)	*gyrA/gyrB*	eubacteria	negative supercoiling	A_2B_2
Topo IV (II)	*parC/parE*	eubacteria	decatenation	C_2E_2
Topo II (II)	*top2 (top2α, top2β)*	eukaryotes and T-even phages	decatenation/catenation relaxation of (+,–) supercoils	homodimer

residue from the phosphate. Camptothecin presumably interferes with this reaction by blocking the rejoining step.[7,38] Such a blockage results in the accumulation of a reversible enzyme-camptothecin-DNA ternary complex, termed the cleavable complex.[7] Denaturation of this cleavable complex with a strong protein denaturant such as SDS or alkali results in the formation of an enzyme-linked DNA break. Biochemical studies have suggested that camptothecin may bind only to the topoisomerase I-DNA complex but not to the enzyme or DNA.[39]

Studies using the purified topoisomerase I has also revealed that some of the camptothecin derivatives (e.g., 10,11-methylenedioxy-camptothecin and 9-amino-10,11-methlenedioxy-camptothecin) are more potent inhibitors.[12,15] In addition, the 20[S] form of camptothecin is active, but the 20[R] counterpart is completely inactive, indicating a stereo-specific receptor site on topoisomerase I.[12]

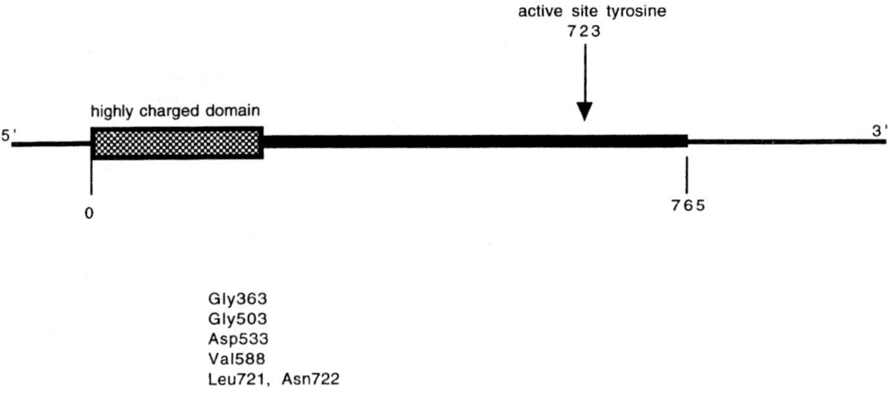

Figure 2 Human DNA topoisomerase I cDNA. The amino acid residues listed represent sites of mutations that can lead to camptothecin resistance.

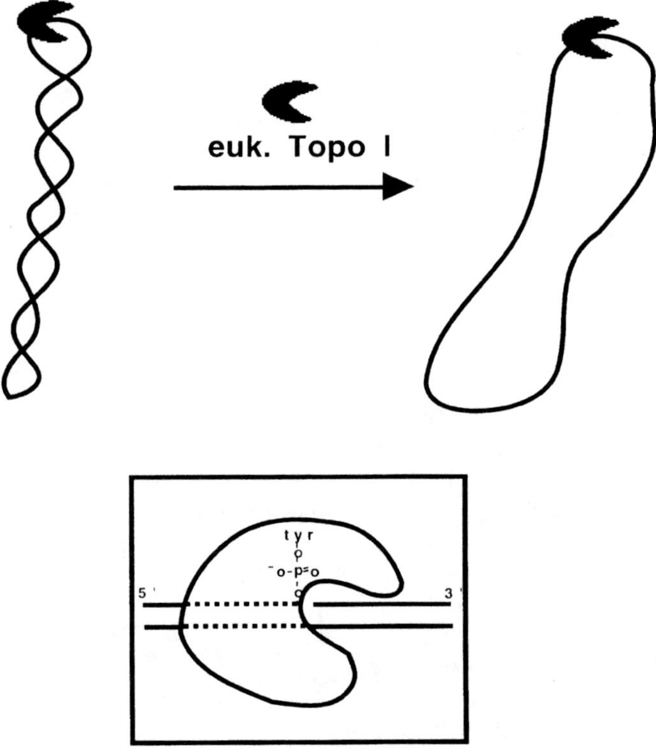

Figure 3 Relaxation by mammalian DNA topoisomerase I.

V. MECHANISM OF CELL KILLING

Overwhelming evidence has supported the view that cell killing by camptopthecin is due to the formation of topoisomerase I-camptothecin-DNA cleavable complexes.[40,41] Inhibition of the relaxation activity of topoisomerase I is apparently inconsequential as far as cell killing is concerned.[40] A yeast *top*1 deletion strain was shown to be highly resistant to camptothecin. However, expression of human topoisomerase I in this yeast *top*1 strain dramatically sensitized yeast toward camptothecin.[40] It is therefore predicted that tumor cells with high levels of topoisomerase I should be more sensitive to camptothecin and vice versa. Indeed, several camptothecin-resistant tumor cell lines have been shown to have reduced expression of topoisomerase I.[42,43]

The reversibility of topoisomerase I-camptothecin-DNA cleavable complexes has raised the question of how tumor cells are killed by these reversible complexes. Studies with replication inhibitors have shown that transient inhibition of DNA replication during camptothecin treatment can completely abolish camptothecin cytotoxicity, suggesting an involvement of active DNA replication in camptothecin cytotoxicity.[8,44,45] Studies in a cell-free SV40 replication system have further suggested a fork collision model for camptothecin cytotoxicity.[8] In this model, the interaction between the replication fork and the topoisomerase I-camptothecin-DNA cleavable complex is presumed to be the lethal event and results in at least three detectable changes: irreversible arrest of DNA replication forks, double-strand DNA breaks at the forks, and the conversion of reversible cleavable complexes into cleaved complexes (see Figure 1). Presumably, one of several of these changes is the trigger for cell death and G2 cell cycle arrest.[8,46] Interestingly, the

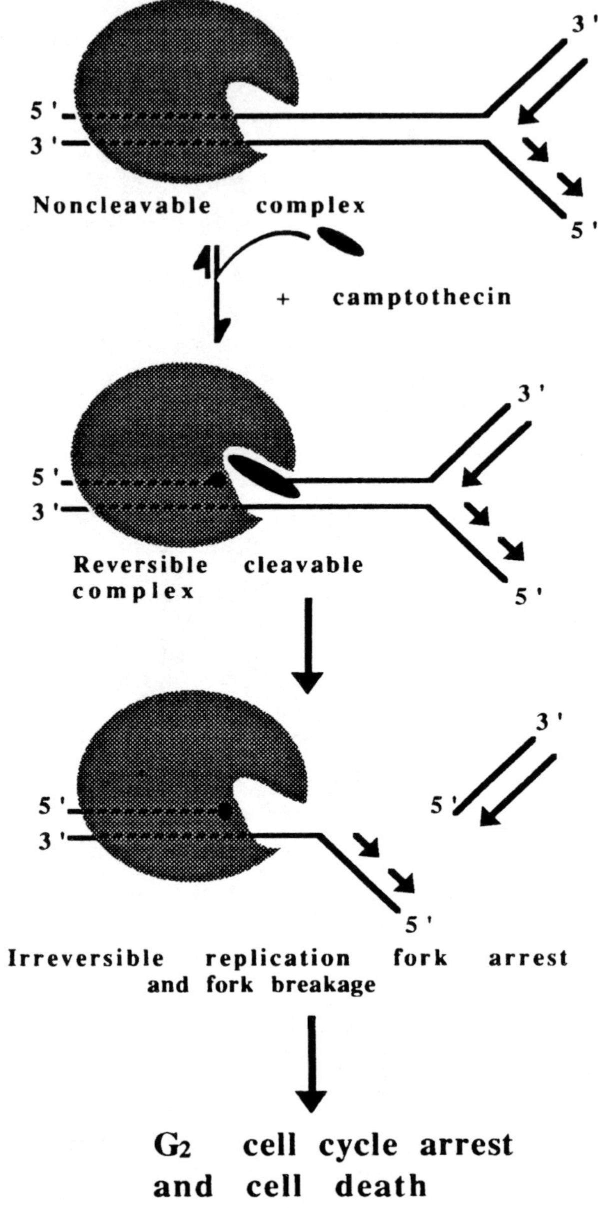

Figure 4 Mechanism of cell killing by camptothecins.

polarity of the topoisomerase I cleavable complex appears to be critical. The formation of the cleavable complex on the parental strand that is complementary to the leading but not lagging strand of DNA synthesis has been shown to lead to the lethal collision.

Studies in *Saccharomyces cerevisiae* have shown that *rad52* mutations can confer hypersensitivity to camptothecin,VP-16 and m-AMSA.[40,47] *rad52* Is known to be involved in the repair of double-strand DNA breaks in yeast.[47] These results, which are consistent with results obtained in mammalian cells, suggest the involvement of a DNA repair mechanism in cell killing by topoisomerase drugs and that DNA double-strand breaks may be central to cell killing by topoisomerase drugs.

Camptothecin has also been shown to induce differentiation of human promyelocytic leukemia cells HL60, human promonocytic leukemia cells U-937, and human leukaemic cells K562.[48-50] Induction of *c-fos* and *c-jun* mRNAs is also observed.[49,51] However, whether these responses are related to S-phase cytotoxicity of camptothecin is not known.

IV. DRUG RESISTANCE

Camptothecin and its noncharged derivatives have been shown to be highly effective against many human solid tumor xenografts in nude mice, including the highly refractory human colon tumors. [36,52,53] This unexpected result has led to an investigation of camptothecin's ability to overcome drug resistance in tumors. Studies using MDR1-overexpressing cells have demonstrated that camptothecin and its noncharged derivatives can overcome MDR1-mediated resistance.[54] However, the positively charged camptothecin derivative, topotecan, is moderately sensitive to MDR1.[54] Whether the ability of camptothecin to overcome MDR1-mediated resistance is responsible for its broad spectrum antitumor activity remains to be answered. The impressive ability of camptothecin to overcome MDR1-mediated resistance has been attributed to the rapid passive diffusion of camptothecin, the lack of an interaction with MDR1, or a combination of both.[54]

Mutant cell lines which are made resistant to camptothecin have been isolated.[41-43,55] Mutations in the structural gene of topoisomerase I, decrease in topoisomerase I levels, and lengthened cell cycle time in these mutant cell lines have been observed. The most well-characterized mutant topoisomerase I is from the CPT-resistant human acute lymphoblastic leukemia cell line (CPT-K5).[41,56] Among the two mutations found in the cDNA of the topoisomerase I gene from CPT-K5 cells, both are aspartic acid to glycine changes; the change at residue 533 is probably responsible for resistance to camptothecin.[56] Recent studies on the purified mutant topoisomerase I from CPT-K5 cells have suggested that the alteration on the affinity between the mutant topoisomerase I and DNA is one feature of the mutant enzyme which may be responsible for the mutant enzyme's resistance toward camptothecin.[57] Studies in camptothecin-resistant Chinese hamster cell lines have also demonstrated that a single substitution of serine for Gly505 (corresponding to Gly503 in the human enzyme) results in camptothecin resistance.[55,58]

Yeast has been established as a useful genetic system for studying topoisomerase drugs.[40] Mutations (I725R, N726A) near the active site tyrosine (#727 of the yeast topoisomerase I) have been shown to confer camptothecin resistance. Similar mutations (L721R, N722A) in the human enzyme also result in camptothecin resistance.[59] These mutations occur naturally in *vaccinia* topoisomerase I which is camptothecin-resistant.[17] A mutation (G363C) distal to the active site tyrosine (#723 of the human topoisomerase I) has also been identified on the human enzyme in the yeast system.[58] A summary of the various mutations which are known to confer camptothecin resistance is shown in Figure 2.

VII. CONCLUSIONS

Studies of camptothecin have established the potential of DNA topoisomerase I as a new therapeutic target for cancer chemotherapy. Additional topoisomerase I inhibitors are likely to emerge in the future for clinical development. Already, several new topoisomerase I inhibitors have been reported, including some DNA minor groove binding drugs.[60-62] The success of camptothecin in treating solid tumors in animal models is quite encouraging. The biochemistry of camptothecin action has been significantly advanced. It is expected that studies of camptothecin will lead to a better understanding of the antitumor action of antitumor drugs in general as well as development of new and improved therapy for cancers.

REFERENCES

1. **Bosmann, H. B.,** Camptothecin inhibits macromolecular synthesis in mammalian cells but not in isolated mitochondria or *E. coli. Biochem. Biophy Res. Comm.* 41:1412-1420 (1970).
2. **Kessel, D., Bosmann, H. B., and Lohr, K.,** Camptothecin effects on DNA synthesis in murine leukemia cells. *Biochim. Biophys. Acta* 269:210-216 (1972).
3. **Horwitz, S. B., Chang, C.-K., and Grollman, A. P.,** Studies on camptothecin: Effects on nucleic acid and protein synthesis. *Mol. Pharm.* 7:632-644 (1971).
4. **Horwitz, M. S. and Horwitz, S. B.,** Intracellular degradation of hela and adenovirus type 2 DNA induced by camptothecin. *Biochem. Biophys. Res. Comm.* 45:723-727 (1971).
5. **Li, L. H., Fraser, T. J., Olin, E. J., and Bhuyan, B. K.,** Action of camptothecin on mammalian cells in culture. *Cancer Res.* 32:2643-2650 (1972).
6. **Horwitz, S. B. and Horwitz, M. S.,** Effects of camptothecin on the breakage and repair of DNA during the cell cycle. *Cancer Res.* 33:2834-2836 (1973).
7. **Hsiang, Y.-H., Hertzberg, R., Hecht, S., and Liu, L. F.,** Camptothecin induces protein-linked DNA breaks via mammalian DNA topoisomerase I. *J. Biol. Chem.* 260:14873-14878 (1985).
8. **Hsiang, Y.-H., Lihou, M. G., and Liu, L. F.,** Arrest of replication forks by drug-stabilized topoisomerase 1-DNA cleavable complexes as a mechanism of cell killing by camptothecin. *Cancer Res.* 49:5077-5082 (1989).
9. **Horwitz, S. B., Chang, C.-K., and Grollman, A. P.,** Antiviral action of camptothecin. *Antimicro. Agents and Chemo.* 2:395-401 (1972).
10. **Shuman, S., Golder, M., and Moss, B.,** Characterization of *vaccinia* virus DNA topoisomerase I expressed in *Escherichia coli. J. Biol. Chem.* 263:16401-16407 (1988).
11. **Gupta, M., Zhu, C. X., and Tse, D. Y.,** An engineered mutant of *vaccinia* virus DNA topoisomerase I is sensitive to the anti-cancer drug camptothecin. *J. Biol. Chem.* 267:24177-24180 (1992).
12. **Jaxel, C., Kohn, K. W., Wani, M. C., Wall, M. E., and Pommier, Y.,** Structure-activity study of the actions of camptothecin derivatives on mammalian topoisomerase I: Evidence for a specific receptor site and a relation to antitumor activity. *Cancer Res.* 49:1465-1469 (1989).
13. **Wani, M. C., Nicholas, A. W., Manikumar, G., and Wall, M. E.,** Plant antitumor agents. 25. Total synthesis and antileukemic activity of ring A-substituted camptothecin analogues. Structure-activity correlations. *J. Med. Chem.* 30:1774-1779 (1987).
14. **Wani, M. C., Rommam, P. E., Lindley, J. T., and Wall, M. E.,** Plant antitumor agents. 18. Synthesis and biological activity of camptothecin analogues. *J. Med. Chem.* 23:554-560 (1980).
15. **Hsiang, Y.-H., Liu, L. F., Wall, M. E., Wani, N. C., Nicholas, A. W., Manikumar, G., Kirschenbaum, S., Silber, R., and Potmesil, M.,** DNA topoisomerase I-mediated DNA cleavage and cytotoxicity of camptothecin analogs. *Cancer Res.* 49:4385-4389 (1989).
16. **Liu, L. F., Liu, C. C., and Alberts, B. M.,** Type II DNA topoisomerases. Enzymes that can unknot a topologically knotted DNA molecule via a reversible double-strand break. *Cell* 19:697-707 (1980).

17. **Brown, P. O. and Cozzarelli, N. R.,** A sign inversion mechanism for enzymatic supercoiling of DNA. *Science* 206:1081-1083 (1979).

18. **Liu, L. F.,** DNA topoisomerases — enzymes that catalyze the breaking and rejoining of DNA. *CRC Review of Biochem.* 15, 1-24 (1983).

19. **D'Arpa, P., Machlin, P. S., Ratrie, H., III, Rothfield, N. F., Cleveland, D. W., and Earnshaw, W. C.,** cDNA cloning of human DNA topoisomerase I: Catalytic activity of a 67.7-kDa carboxyl-terminal fragment. *Proc. Natl. Acad. Sci. U.S.A.* 85:2543-2547 (1988).

20. **Pflugfelder, M. T., Liu, L. F., Liu, A. A., Tewey, K. M., Whang-Peng, J., Knutsen, T., Huebner, K., Croce, C. M., and Wang, J. C.,** Cloning and sequencing of cDNA encoding human DNA topoisomerase II and localization of the gene to chromosome 17q21-21. *Proc. Natl. Acad. Sci. U.S.A.* 85:7177-7181 (1988).

21. **Chung, T. D. Y., Drake, F. H., Tan, K. B., Per, S. R., Crooke, S. T., and Mirabelli, C. K.,** Characterization and immunological identification of cDNA clones encoding two human topoisomerase II isozymes. *Proc. Natl. Acad. Sci. U.S.A.* 86:9431-9435 (1989).

22. **Liu, L. F.,** DNA topoisomerase poisons as antitumor drugs. *Ann. Rev. Biochem.* 58:351-375 (1989).

23. **D'Arpa, P. and Liu, L. F.,** Topoisomerase-targeting antitumor drugs. *Biochim. Biophys. Acta.* 989:163-177 (1989).

24. **Hsiang, Y.-H. and Liu, L. F.,** Identification of mammalian DNA topoisomerase I as an intracellular target of the anticancer drug camptothecin. *Cancer Res.* 48:1722-1726 (1988).

25. **Champoux, J. J. and Dulbecco, R.,** An activity from mammalian cells that untwists superhelical DNA — A possible swivel for DNA replication. *Proc. Natl. Acad. Sci. U.S.A.* 69:143-146 (1972).

26. **Liu, L. F. and Miller, K. G.,** Eukaryotic DNA topoisomerases. Two forms of type I DNA topoisomerases from HeLa cell nuclei. *Proc. Natl. Acad. Sci. U.S.A.* 78:3487-3491 (1981).

27. **D'Arpa, P., Machlin, P. S., Ratrie, H., III, Rothfield, N. F., Cleveland, D. W., and Earnshaw, W. C.,** cDNA cloning of human DNA topoisomerase I: Catalytic activity of a 67.7-kDa carboxyl-terminal fragment. *Proc. Natl. Acad. Sci. U.S.A.* 85:2543-2547 (1988).

28. **Juan, C.-C., Hwang, J., Liu, A. A., Whang-Peng, J., Knutsen, T., Huebner, K., Croce, C. M., Zhang, H., Wang, J. C., and Liu, L. F.,** Human DNA topoisomerase I is encoded by a single-copy gene that maps to chromosome region 20q12-13.2. *Proc. Natl. Acad. Sci. U.S.A.* 85:8910-8913 (1988).

29. **Yang, L., Wold, M. S., Li, J. J., Kelly, T. J., and Liu, L. F.,** Roles of DNA topoisomerases in SV40 DNA replication *in vitro. Proc. Natl. Acad. Sci. U.S.A.* 84:950-954 (1987).

30. **Liu, L. F. and Wang, J. C.,** Supercoiling of the DNA template during transcription. *Proc. Natl. Acad. Sci. U.S.A.* 84:7024-7027 (1987).

31. **Zhang, H., Wang, J. C., and Liu, L. F.,** Involvement of DNA topoisomerase I in transcription of human ribosomal RNA genes. *Proc. Natl. Acad. Sci. U.S.A.* 85:1060-1064 (1988).

32. **Merino, A., Madden, K. R., Lane, W. S., Champoux, J. J., and Reinberg, D.,** DNA topoisomerase I is involved in both repression and activation of transcription. *Nature* 365:227-232 (1993).

33. **Lynn, R. M., Bjornsti, M. A., Caron, P. R., and Wang, J. C.,** Peptide sequencing and site-directed mutagenesis identify tyrosine-727 as the active site tyrosine of *Saccharomyces cerevisiae* DNA topoisomerase-I. *Proc. Nat'l Acad. Sci. U.S.A.* 86:3559-3563 (1989).

34. **Hwong, C. L., Chen, M. S., and Hwang, J.,** Phorbol ester transiently increases topoisomerase I mRNA levels in human skin fibroblasts. *J. Biol. Chem.* 264:14923-14926 (1989).

35. **Hwong, C. L., Chen, C. Y., Shang, H. F., and Hwang, J.,** Increased synthesis and degradation of DNA topoisomerase I during the initial phase of human T-lymphocyte proliferation. *J. Biol. Chem.* 268:18982-18986 (1993).

36. **Giovanella, B. C., J. S. Stehlin, W. E., Wall, M. C., Wani, A. W., Nicholas, L., Liu, L. F., Silber, R., and Potmesil, M.,** DNA topoisomerase I-targeted chemotherapy of human colon cancer in xenografts. *Science* 246:1046-1048 (1989).

37. **Champoux, J. J.,** DNA is linked to the rat liver nicking-closing enzyme by a phosphodiester bond to tyrosine. *J. Biol. Chem.* 256:4805-4809 (1981).

38. **Porter, S. E. and Champoux, J. J.,** The basis for camptothecin enhancement of DNA breakage by eukaryotic topoisomerase I. *Nucl. Acids Res.* 17:8521-8532 (1989).

39. **Hertzberg, R. P., Caranfa, M. J., and Hecht, S. M.,** On the mechanism of topoisomerase I inhibition by camptothecin — Evidence for binding to an enzyme DNA complex. *Biochem.* 28:4629-4638 (1989).

40. **Nitiss, J. and Wang, J. C.,** DNA topoisomerase-targeting antitumor drugs can be studied in yeast. *Proc. Natl. Acad. Sci. U.S.A.* 85:7501-7505 (1988).

41. **Andoh, T., Ishii, K., Suzuki, Y., Ikegami, Y., Kusunoki, Y., Takemoto, Y., and Okada, K.,** Characterization of a mammalian mutant with a camptothecin-resistant DNA topoisomerase I. *Proc. Natl. Acad. Sci. U.S.A.* 84:5565-5569 (1987).

42. **Sugimoto, Y., Tsukahara, S., Ohhara, T., Liu, L. F., and Tsuruo, T.,** Elevated expression of DNA topoisomerase II in camptothecin-resistant human tumor cell lines. *Cancer Res.* 50:7962-7965 (1990).

43. **Kanzawa, F., Sugimoto, Y., Minato, K., Kasahara, K., Bungo, M., Nakagawa, K., Fujiwara, Y., Liu, L. F., and Saijo, N.,** Establishment of a camptothecin analogue (CPT-11)-resistant cell line of human non-small cell lung cancer: Characterization and mechanism of resistance. *Cancer Res.* 50:5919-5924 (1990).

44. **Holm, C., Covey, J. M., Kerrigan, D., and Pommier, Y.,** Differential requirement of DNA replication for the cytotoxicity of DNA topoisomerase I and II inhibitors in Chinese hamster DC3F cells. *Cancer Res.* 49:6365-6368 (1989).

45. **D'Arpa, P., Beardmore, C., and Liu, L. F.,** Involvement of nucleic acid synthesis in cell killing mechanisms of topoisomerase poisons. *Cancer Res.* 50:6919-6924 (1990).

46. **Tsao, Y. P., D'Arpa, P., and Liu, L. F.,** The involvement of active DNA synthesis in camptothecin-induced G2 arrest: Altered regulation of p34cdc2/cyclin B. *Cancer Res.* 52:1823-1829 (1992).

47. **Nitiss, J. and Wang, J. C.,** Yeast as a genetic system in the dissection of the mechanism of cell killing by topoisomerase-targeting anticancer drugs. In *DNA Topoisomerase in Cancer,* Potmesil, M. and Kohn, K. W., Eds., Oxford University Press, New York, 77-90 (1991).

48. **Ling, Y. H., Tseng, M. T., and Nelson, J. A.,** Differentiation induction of human promyelocytic leukemia cells by 10-hydroxycamptothecin, a DNA topoisomerase I inhibitor. *Differentiation* 46:135-141 (1991).

49. **Aller, P., Rius, C., Mata, F., Zorrilla, A., Cabanas, C., Bellon, T., and Bernabeu, C.,** Camptothecin induces differentiation and stimulates the expression of differentiation-related genes in U-937 human promonocytic leukemia cells. *Cancer Res.* 52:1245-1251 (1992).

50. **McSheehy, P. M., Gervasoni, M., Lampasona, V., Erba, E., and D'Incalci, M.,** Studies of the differentiation properties of camptothecin in the human leukaemic cells K562. *Eur. J. Cancer* 27:1406-1411 (1991).

51. **Kharbanda, S., Rubin, E., Gunji, H., Hinz, H., Giovanella, B., Pantazis, P., and Kufe, D.,** Camptothecin and its derivatives induce expression of the *c-jun* protooncogene in human myeloid leukemia cells. *Cancer Res.* 51:6636-6642 (1991).

52. **Pantazis, P., Early, J. A., Kozielski, A. J., Mendoza, J. T., Hinz, H. R., and Giovanella, B.,** Regression of human breast carcinoma tumors in immunodeficient mice treated with 9-nitrocamptothecin: Differential response of nontumorigenic and tumorigenic human breast cells *in vitro. Cancer Res.* 53:1577-1582 (1993).

53. **Pantazis, P., Kozielski, A. J., Mendoza, J. T., Early, J. A., Hinz, H. R., and Giovanella, B.,** Camptothecin derivatives induce regression of human ovarian carcinomas grown in nude mice and distinguish between nontumorigenic and tumorigenic cells *in vitro. Int. J. Cancer* 863-871 (1993).

54. **Chen, A. Y., Yu, C., Potmesil, M., Wall, M. E., Wani, M. C., and Liu, L. F.,** Camptothecin overcomes MDR1-mediated resistance in human KB carcinoma cells. *Cancer Res.* 51:6039-6044 (1991).

55. **Tanizawa, A. and Pommier, Y.,** Topoisomerase I alteration in a camptothecin-resistant cell line derived from Chinese hamster DC3F cells in culture. *Cancer Res.* 52:1848-1854 (1992).

56. **Tamura, H., Kohchi, C., Yamada, R., Ikeda, T., Koiwai, O., Patterson, E., Keene, J. D., Okada, K., Kjeldsen, E., Nishikawa, K., and Andoh, T.,** Molecular cloning of a cDNA of a camptothecin-resistant human DNA topoisomerase I and identification of mutation sites. *Nucl. Acids Res.* 19:69-75 (1991).

57. **Gromova, I. I., Kjeldsen, E., Svejstrup, J. Q., Alsner, J., Christiansen, K., and Westergaard, O.,** Characterization of an altered DNA catalysis of a camptothecin-resistant eukaryotic topoisomerase I. *Nucleic Acids Res.* 21:593-600 (1993).

58. **Benedetti, P., Fiorani, P., Capuani, L., and Wang, J. C.,** Camptothecin resistance from a single mutation changing glycine 363 of human DNA topoisomerase I to cysteine. *Cancer Res.* 53:4343-4348 (1993).

59. **Knab, A. M., Fertala, J., and Bjorski, M.-A.,** Mechanisms of camptothecin resistance in yeast DNA topoisomerase I mutants. *J. Biol. Chem.* 268: 22322-22330 (1993).

60. **Chen, A. Y. and Liu, L. F.,** Mechanisms of resistance to topoisomerase inhibitors. In *Cancer Treatment and Research,* Ozols, R. F. and Goldstein, L., Eds., Kluwer Academic Press, Massachusetts, in press.

61. **Yoshinari, T., Yamada, A., Uemura, D., Nomura, K., Arakawa, H., Kojiri, K., Yoshida, E., Suda, H., and Okura, A.,** Induction of topoisomerase I-mediated DNA cleavage by a new indolocarbazole, ED-110. *Cancer Res.* 53:490-494 (1993).

62. **Fujii, N., Yamashita, Y., Saitoh, Y., and Nakano, H.,** Induction of mammalian DNA topoisomerase I-mediated DNA cleavage and DNA winding by bulgarein. *J. Biol. Chem.* 268:13160-13165 (1993).

Camptothecin and Analogs: From Discovery to Clinic

Monroe E. Wall and Mansukh C. Wani

CONTENTS

I. INTRODUCTION

Camptothecin (CPT) (1, Figure 1) is a naturally occurring alkaloid isolated from *Camptotheca acuminata* (Decaisne) (Nyssaceae) which is a native of China found in Szechwan and a number of other provinces.[1] Progress in CPT studies has encountered

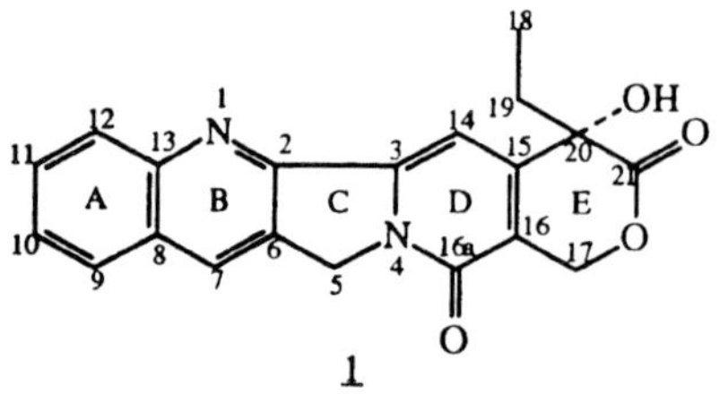

Figure 1 Structures of camptothecin and its analogs discussed in this chapter.

1

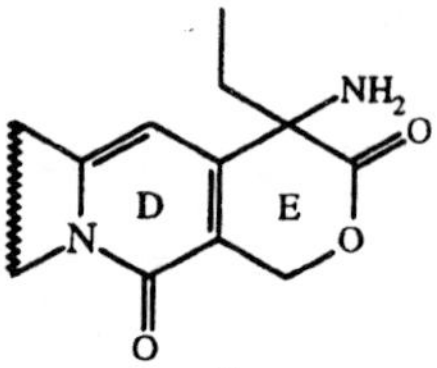

7

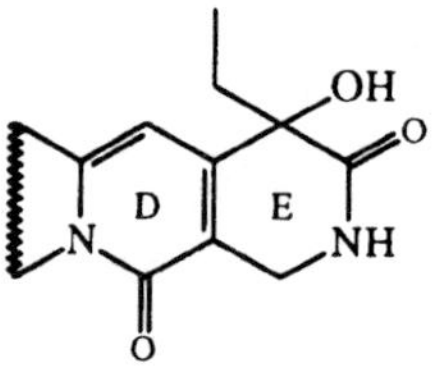

8

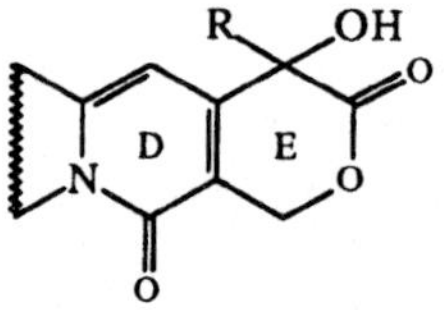

41, R = CH₃, 20(RS)

42, R = CH₂CH₂OH, 20(RS)

43, R = CH₂CH₂Br, 20(RS)

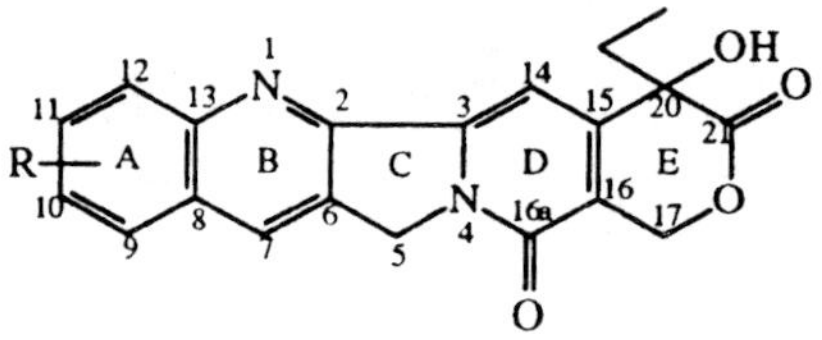

3, R = 10-OH, 20(S)	16, R = 9-Cl, 20(S)	25, R = 9-(CH₂)₂NCH₂-10-OH•HCl
6, R = 9-NH₂-10,11-OCH₂O-, 20(S)	17, R = 10-Cl, 20(S)	26, R = 10,11-OCH₃, 20(RS)
9, R = 9-NH₂, 20(S)	18, R = 9-CH₃, 20(S)	27, R = 10,11-OCH₂O-, 20(RS)
10, R = 10-NH₂, 20(S)	19, R = 11-CN, 20(RS)	28, R = 10,11-OCH₂O-, 20(S)
11, R = 9-NO₂, 20(S)	20, R = 11-OH, 20(RS)	29, R = 9-NH₂-10,11-OCH₂O-, 20(RS)
12, R = 10-NO₂, 20(RS)	21, R = 11-NH₂, 20(RS)	30, R = 9-Cl-10,11-OCH₂O-, 20(S)
13, R = 10-NO₂, 20(S)	22, R = 12-NH₂, 20(S)	31, R = 10,11-O(CH₂)₂O-, 20(RS)
14, R = 9-OH, 20(RS)	23, 9-NO₂-10-OH, 20(S)	32, R = 9,10-OCH₂O-, 20(RS)
15, R = 9-OH, 20(S)	24, 9-NHCOCH₃-10-OH, 20(S)	

many obstacles and vicissitudes since the first attempted introduction of *C. acuminata* into the United States took place more than eighty years ago. The antitumor activity in *C. acuminata* extracts was discovered about thirty-five years ago, and initial abortive clinical trials with CPT sodium salt took place somewhat over twenty years ago.

Much of this information is little known today. Because of the fact that camptothecin and its analogs have again come into prominence and are in active clinical trial for a variety of solid tumors, the interesting but little known history of the early stages of the

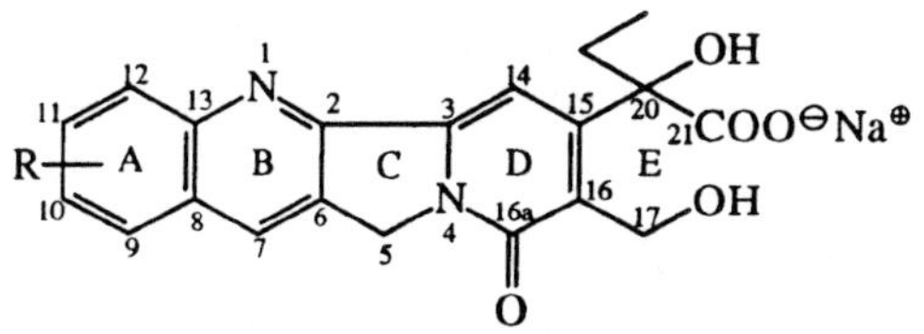

$\underline{2}$, R = H, 20($\underline{S}$)

$\underline{33}$, R = 9-NH_2-10,11-OCH_2O-, 20($\underline{S}$)

$\underline{34}$, R = 10-ONa, 20($\underline{S}$)

$\underline{35}$, R = 9-NH_2, 20($\underline{RS}$)

$\underline{36}$, R = 10,11-OCH_2O-, 20($\underline{RS}$)

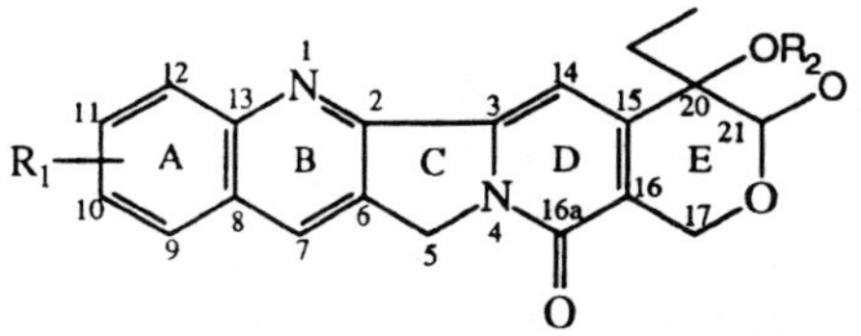

$\underline{37}$, R_1 = 9-$NHCOCH_2NH_2\cdot HCl$, R_2 = H, 20($\underline{RS}$)

$\underline{38}$, R_1 = 9-NH_2, R_2 = $COCH_2NH_2\cdot HCl$, 20($\underline{RS}$)

$\underline{39}$, R_1 = 10-NH_2, R_2 = $COCH_2NH_2\cdot HCl$, 20($\underline{RS}$)

$\underline{40}$, R_1 = 10,11-OCH_2O-, R_2 = $COCH_2NH_2\cdot HCl$, 20($\underline{RS}$)

Figure 1 (continued)

development of CPT will be presented in detail. This will be followed by a concise resume of SAR studies of CPT and analogs, synthetic methods, a correlation of *in vivo* and *in vitro* activities with particular emphasis on topoisomerase I inhibition, and finally a description of the current status of camptothecin and its analogs as therapeutic agents in chemotherapy.

II. DISCOVERY OF CAMPTOTHECIN

A. INTRODUCTION OF *C. ACUMINATA* TO THE UNITED STATES

Probably the most detailed account of taxonomical information and details of the introduction of *C. acuminata* into the United States has been published by Purdue et al.[1] *C. acuminata* is found in several provinces of China, notably Szechwan, and requires frost-free and relatively mild climates for successful growth. On a number of occasions since 1911, seeds were sent to various plant introduction groups in the U.S. In 1934, seeds of *C. acuminata* were received at the USDA Plant Introduction Garden, Beltsville, Maryland. After being slated for discarding, the seeds were found to germinate readily, and a number of plants were grown and sent to various plant introduction gardens of the USDA. Several were received at the Chico, California, Plant Introduction Garden, and by 1950 several of these trees were being grown in that area and elsewhere in California. In 1950, one of us (M.E. Wall) was placed in charge of a program at the Eastern Regional

Research Laboratory (ERRL), USDA, Philadelphia, which had as a major objective the procurement of plants with steroids suitable for the synthesis of cortisone. During the period 1949–1959, thousands of plants were screened for steroids.

The plant collections were conducted by botanists under the auspices of the Plant Introduction Division of the USDA. The plants were collected and meticulously identified before shipping to the ERRL. This joint effort of chemists and botanists proved to be a good model for future programs. Indeed, it firmly established the fact that the close cooperation between chemists and botanists was required for a successful natural product discovery program. The survey included not only quantitative data for steroidal sapogenins but also qualitative analysis for sterols, alkaloids, tannins, and flavonoids. A large number of the alcoholic extracts of plants which were unusual or which had received little chemical study in the past were stored and saved.

B. ANTITUMOR ACTIVITY OF EXTRACTS OF *C. ACUMINATA*

In addition to screening the plants collected for various chemical constituents, the extracts were also tested biologically for antibiotic, antitumor, and antiviral activity. In 1957, Dr. Wall was visited by the late Dr. Jonathan Hartwell, Cancer Chemotherapy National Service Center (CCNSC) of the National Cancer Institute (NCI). After discussions with Dr. Hartwell (who was considered by many natural products scientists to be the pioneer worker in the field of plant antitumor constituents), it was agreed to send him 1000 alcoholic plant extracts for testing for antitumor activity. Almost one year later, the astonishing result was transmitted to Wall that of all the extracts submitted, only the extract of *C. acuminata* had high activity in the CA755 assay then used as one of the NCI standard *in vivo* assay systems.[2] Subsequently, the crude *C. acuminata* extracts were also found to be very active in a mouse leukemia assay (L1210). For administrative reasons, it was impossible for Dr. Wall to pursue the isolation of 1 at the ERRL. In 1960, Wall established a natural products laboratory at the Research Triangle Institute with the express purpose of isolating antitumor principles from plants and/or other natural products. In 1961, with support from the NCI, fractionation of *C. acuminata* was initiated. For this purpose, sizeable samples of the wood and bark from *C. acuminata* grown at Chico, California, became available.

C. FRACTIONATION OF *C. ACUMINATA*
1. Extraction of Plant Material

Figure 2 presents details of the extraction procedure. In brief, the sample was subjected to a continuous hot extraction with heptane. The residual marc was then subjected to continuous extraction with hot 95% ethanol. After concentration of the ethanol extract, the residue was partitioned between chloroform and water. As shown in Figure 2, the various extracts were assayed for activity in L1210 mouse leukemia. This assay involves a life prolongation evaluation. If the control animals live 10 days and the animals receiving the test material live 12.5 days, that would be a T/C of 125% which would be regarded as the borderline for a statistically significant result by NCI protocol.[3] It was evident that the activity is concentrated in the chloroform-soluble fractions. This procedure and subsequent purification procedures were one of the first examples of fractionation of natural product extracts according to bioactivity rather than a specific search for a specific constituent.

Most of the chloroform phase (Figure 2) after concentration was subjected to an 11-stage preparative Craig countercurrent distribution as shown in Table 1. In this very simple use of the Craig methodology, the partition was carried out in large separatory funnels using a chloroform-carbontetrachloride-methanol-water partition system with the ratios shown in Table 1. All of the fractions were analyzed by both the *in vivo* L1210 mouse life prolongation assay and by a 9KB *in vitro* cytotoxicity assay. There was

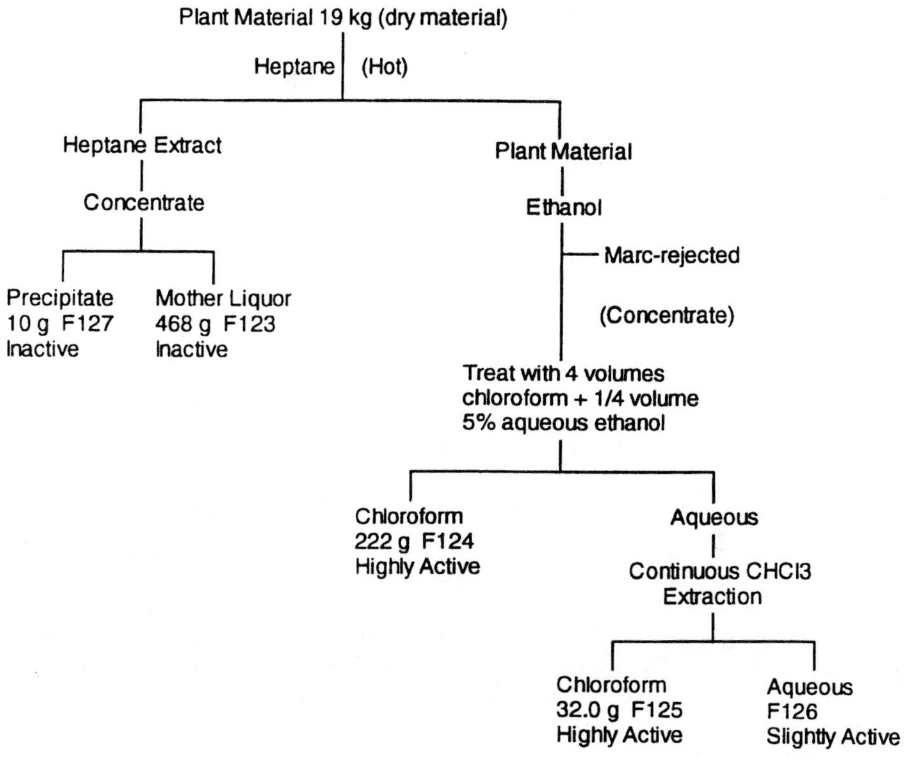

Figure 2 Fractionation of *Camptotheca acuminata.*

reasonable correlation between the two assays. Tubes 2–6 were judged to contain the most active material. It should be kept in mind that in the *in vivo* life prolongation assay, it is the combination of the lowest dose with the largest T/C activity which is the basis for selecting active fractions. In the cytotoxicity assay, it is simply the lowest ED_{50} dose which inhibits the growth of the 9KB cells. Thus, about 80% of the total weight was removed while concentrating the most active fractions in 20% of the original weight of the chloroform extracts. By comparison with a pure sample obtained later, but again given the standard L1210 assay (cf. K-128 in Table 1), it can be estimated that the most active fractions contained between 1–2% of the active compound. It should be noted that 9KB activity was reasonably correlated with the L1210 assay.

2. Isolation of Camptothecin

When fractions 2–6 were combined and the solvent partially concentrated, a yellow precipitate was formed and collected by filtration. This material was subsequently further

Table 1   Craig countercurrent distribution of the chloroform extract from Figure 2

NSC No.	Tube No.	Wt. Fraction (g)	Dose (mg/kg)[a]	T/C	9KB
FO98	—[b]	—	125	153	<1.0
FO99	1	21.5	250	179	5.3
FO100	2	8.7	62.5	201	0.8
FO101	3	7.2	62.5	201	0.5
FO102	4	6.9	31.2	206	0.09
FO103	5	7.6	31.2	156	0.3
FO104	6	7.2	31.2	198	0.5
FO105	7	9.3	31.2	160	<1.0
FO106	8	11.5	250	172	0.5
FO107	9	16.1	250	148	4.3
FO108	10	19.2	250	96	33.0
FO109	11	62.7	250	100	>100.0
K128 (Camptothecin)	—	—	0.5	163	0.7

[a]Starting material. [b]Dose at which maximum T/C in L1210 was observed.

purified by chromatography on a silica gel column and crystallization. The pure compound was very active in L1210. Doses as low as 0.5 mg/kg gave an appreciable life prolongation. A dose of 4 mg/kg was the maximum tolerated dose prior to occurrence of toxicity.

3. Physical Properties

Some of the major physical properties of CPT ($\underline{1}$) are listed here. The compound was a high melting substance, with a molecular weight of 348.111, obtained by high resolution mass spectrometry, corresponding to the formula $C_{20}H_{16}N_2O_4$. It gave an intense blue fluorescence under UV and was optically active $[\alpha]^{25}_D$, + 31.3°. The compound gave the following qualitative reactions: negative phenol ($FeCl_3$), indole, Dragendorff, and Mayer tests. No crystalline salts could be obtained with a variety of acids. The compound could not be methylated with diazomethane or dimethyl sulphate under a variety of conditions. The compound did not react with bicarbonate or carbonate but could be quantitatively converted to the sodium salt ($\underline{2}$) with sodium hydroxide at room temperature. On acidification, the sodium salt regenerated CPT. The parent compound, however, is extremely water insoluble and, indeed, is insoluble in virtually all organic compounds except dimethylsulfoxide in which it exhibits moderate solubility. Other spectral properties have been presented in detail.[4]

D. STRUCTURE OF CAMPTOTHECIN

It was found that camptothecin can be readily converted to an acetate and a chloroacetate. The chloroacetate was converted to the corresponding iodoacetate by treatment with sodium iodide in acetone. The iodoacetate crystallized in orthorhombic crystals suitable for x-ray analysis. This was carried out by Drs. A. T. McPhail and G. A. Sim, then in the Department of Chemistry, University of Illinois. The structures of camptothecin and the corresponding sodium salt are shown in Figure 1. This structure was completely in accord with ultraviolet, infrared, NMR, and mass spectral data. The structure is unique. Camptothecin has been shown to be related to the indole alkaloids, and the 6-membered ring B and a 5-membered ring C are formed by a ring expansion/ring contraction sequence of reactions. The pentacyclic ring structure is highly unsaturated. Some of the unique structural features involve the presence in ring E of an α-hydroxylactone system and in ring D a conjugated pyridone moiety. CPT has only one asymmetric carbon, C20, with the 20(S) configuration.

III. BIOLOGICAL ACTIVITY OF CAMPTOTHECIN AND ITS SODIUM SALT

As stated previously, CPT was remarkably active in the life prolongation of mice injected with L1210 leukemia cells, showing activity in doses between 0.5–4.0 mg/kg. It showed activity of a similar order in the life prolongation assay for mouse P388 leukemia. The compound was also very active in the inhibition of animal solid tumors that were being studied at this early stage, including the Walker 5WM tumor which was completely inhibited by CPT.[5-7]

As stated previously, on treatment of CPT with sodium hydroxide under mild reaction conditions, the lactone in ring E is hydrolyzed forming the sodium salt (2). It was not until much later that it was shown by definitive comparative studies that this compound was only one-tenth as active as CPT in the P388 mouse leukemia assay.[7] The CPT sodium salt (2) received early clinical trial.[8-11] This topic is reviewed in detail by Franco Muggia, Chapter 3.

IV. ANALOG SYNTHESIS AND EFFECT OF SUBSTITUENTS ON BIOLOGICAL ACTIVITIES

A. INITIAL SAR STUDIES

Camptothecin (1) and 10-hydroxy-20(S)-CPT (3)[5] were isolated in sufficient quantity to permit studies on modifications of the α-hydroxy and lactone moieties in ring E and to obtain information on the effect of substitution in ring A. These studies have been described in detail.[6] In summary, the α-hydroxylactone in ring E was found to be an absolute requirement for *in vitro* and *in vivo* activity of CPT and its analogs, and the introduction of a hydroxyl group in ring A potentiated the activity in respect to CPT.

B. TOTAL SYNTHESIS OF CAMPTOTHECIN AND ANALOGS

After our report on the structure of 1, many novel total syntheses of 1 were reported. However, none of these numerous early syntheses, including one from our laboratory, provided 1 in adequate yields, nor were they sufficiently versatile to permit analog synthesis (cf. Reference 13 for a comprehensive review).

1. Friedlander Synthesis

Improved procedures for the total synthesis of CPT and its analogs developed at RTI involving the Friedlander reaction of properly substituted o-aminobenzaldehydes or acetophenones with a tricyclic synthon have permitted studies of the effects of modifications in rings A, D and E.[7,14-18] Figure 3 presents the application of this synthesis to a wide variety of A-ring substituted CPT analogs, to the synthesis of a tetracyclic CPT analog (4)[18] and to the synthesis of a ring D benzo analog (5).[14]

2. Stereochemistry at C20

As discussed previously, the C20 α-hydroxyl moiety is required for *in vitro* and *in vivo* activity of CPT. Recent studies have provided even greater information on the specificity required in this system. Resolution of the (RS) tricyclic synthon (Figure 4) into the (S) and (R) components enabled us to prepare 20(S)-1 and the corresponding 20(R)-CPT.[19] The stereochemistry of the naturally occurring alkaloid is 20(S). The 20(R) form is inactive in the *in vivo* L1210 mouse leukemia assay and *in vitro* assays.[19] Thus, not only

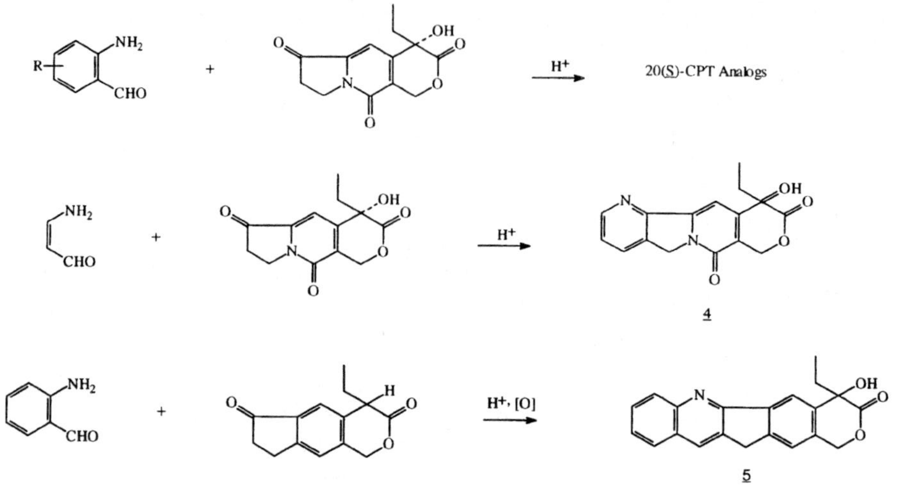

Figure 3 Friedlander condensation of an appropriately substituted *o*-aminobenzaldehyde with a tricyclic synthon.

is the C20-α-hydroxyl moiety required, but correct specific stereochemistry at C20 is also an absolute necessity for *in vitro* cytotoxicity, inhibition of T-1 activity, and *in vivo* antitumor activity.[20-22] Figure 5 shows the synthesis of a highly active compound, 9-amino-10,11-methylenedioxy-20(S)-CPT(6) by the Friedlander synthesis.[18] This compound is exceptionally active at very low dose levels (<1.5 mg/kg) in mouse L1210 leukemia, shows high T-1 inhibition in vitro, and recently has shown strong inhibition *in vitro* of resistant human chronic lymphocytic leukemia cells (see Chapter 4).

3. Effect of Substitution of Nitrogen for Oxygen in Ring E

Recent studies from our laboratory have shown that not only must the correct C20 stereochemistry be present for activity, but that the oxygen of the C20 hydroxyl moiety and the oxygen in the lactone ring E cannot be replaced by nitrogen.[14] Thus, 20(RS)-amino-CPT 7 and the 20(S)-lactam analog 8 (Figure 1) are inactive both *in vitro* and *in vivo*.[14]

The lack of activity of the 20-amino analog may be due to the fact that hydrogen bonding to the C21 carbonyl moiety in ring E is weaker than is the case when the C20 hydroxyl moiety is present. As a consequence, the C21 carbonyl in the amino analog 7 is less positively charged and hence is less susceptible to nucleophilic attack. The inactivity of the lactam 8 is readily explicable since lactams are much less reactive than lactones. It seems increasingly apparent that one of the major features of the biological activity of the CPT molecule is the chemical reactivity of the α-hydroxy-lactone moiety towards nucleophiles. For example, 1 readily forms carboxylic salts in the presence of bases or forms amides by reaction with amines.[4] The reactions are reversible, and hence one can postulate a readily reversible reaction involving the lactone carbonyl and a nucleophilic group or an enzyme or enzyme-DNA complex.

4. Ring A Analogs

The synthetic scheme shown in Figure 3 for the synthesis of CPT has also permitted the preparation of many ring A analogs by suitable manipulation of the o-aminobenzaldehyde synthon. Initially, many of the compounds prepared had the 20(RS) stereochemistry at C20.[7,15-17] Potencies of these compounds were lower than those of the corresponding

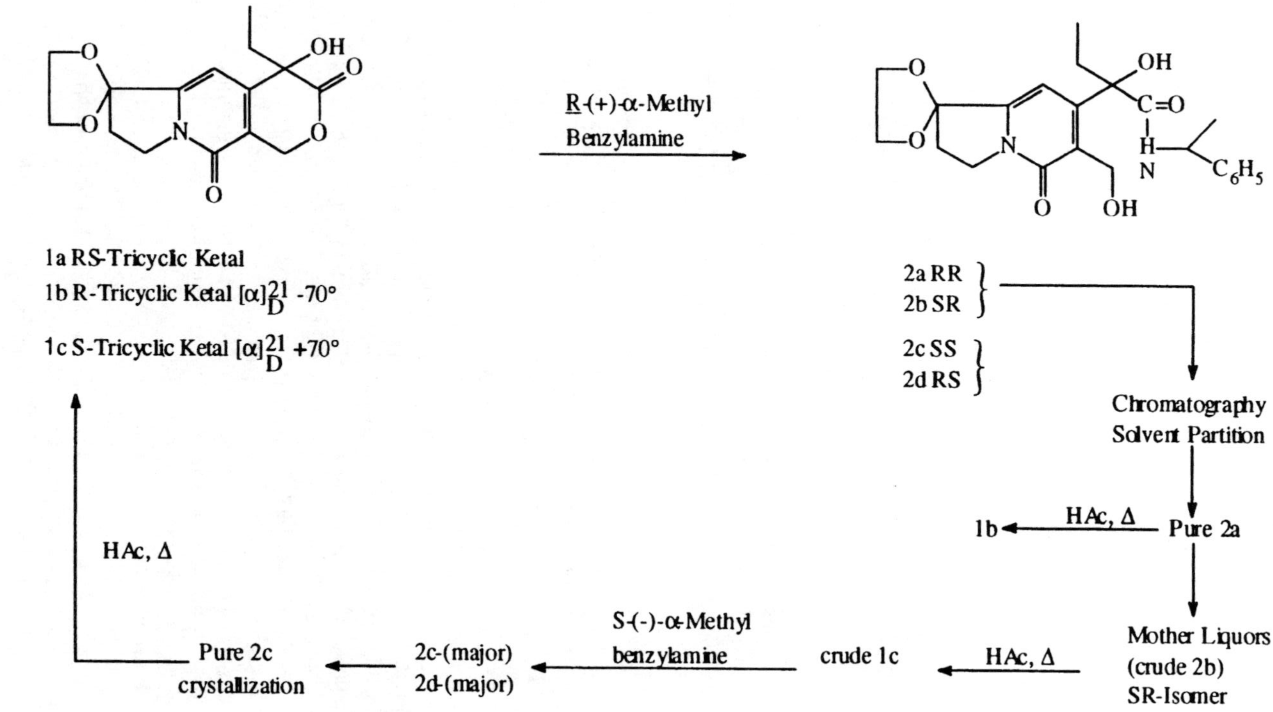

Figure 4 Resolution of 20(RS)-tricyclic synthon.

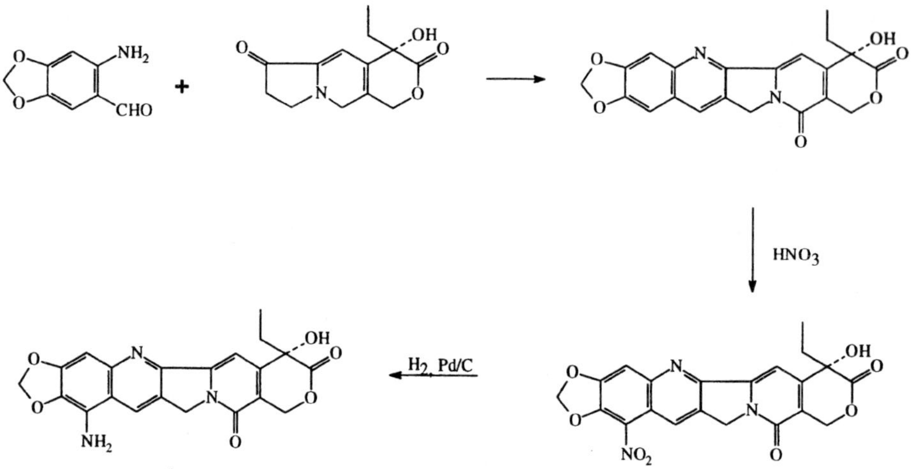

Figure 5 Synthesis of 9-amino-10,11-methylenedioxy-20(S)-camptothecin.

20(S) analogs. Thus, for example, in the mouse P-388 leukemia life prolongation assay, 20(RS)- 1 was found to have a T/C of 200 at 8 mg/kg, whereas in the case of 20(S)-(1), the same activity was found at a dose of 4 mg/kg.[7] The availability of the (S)- and (R)- tricyclic synthons[19] (Figure 3) have permitted the preparation of a number of 20(S)- and 20(R)- analogs of (1).[18] As will be shown subsequently, 20(S)-CPT analogs always exhibit greater potency than the corresponding 20(RS) compounds *in vitro* and *in vivo* (cf. Section VI).

Modification of ring A has yielded many compounds with a wide range of *in vitro* and *in vivo* activity, from exceptionally active to inactive[15-18] (cf.Tables 2, 3). As we will show in subsequent sections, inactivity or loss of activity may result from several factors.

5. Effect of Substitution at C9 and C10

Substitution at C9 or C10 by an amino group leads to compounds with considerably greater *in vivo* activity than is found with the corresponding parent compound 1.[16-17] Thus, both 9-amino-20(S)-CPT (9) and the corresponding 10-amino-20(S) analog (10) are very active compounds in the *in vivo* life prolongation assay for murine L1210 leukemia (Table 2). The 10-amino-20(RS) analog also shows high activity: 9- or 10-nitro-CPT analogs are also active. Thus, the 9-nitro-20(S) analog (11), the corresponding 10-nitro-20(RS) analog (12), and the 10-nitro-20(S) analog (13) have excellent activity *in vivo* (albeit at a considerably higher dose level than corresponding 9- or 10-amino analogs). Although at present there is no experimental proof available that reduction of the nitro substituent to the corresponding amino group occurs *in vivo*, the nitro compounds 11 and 13 may be pro drugs for the corresponding amino analogs 9 and 10.

We have shown previously that 10-hydroxy-20(S)-CPT (3) has excellent life prolongation activity in both L1210 and P-388 murine leukemia.[7,16,17] Rather surprisingly, in view of the high activity *in vivo* (L-1210) and *in vitro* (T-1 inhibition) shown by the 9- and 10-amino analogs (9) and (10), and by the 10-hydroxy analog (3), both the 20(RS) and 20(S) 9-hydroxy analogs (14) and (15), respectively, were weakly active *in vivo* and *in vitro* (cf. Tables 2 and 3).[18]

Table 2 **L1210 mouse leukemia life prolongation by water-insoluble CPT analogs**[a]

Compound	Dose Regimen[b]	Highest Active Dose, mg/Kg (%T/C)[c]	Active Dose Range (mg/kg)	KE[d]	Cures	Toxic Dose mg/kg
20($\underline{S}$)-CPT $\underline{1}$	Q04DX02	12(250)	5.3–12	4.8	1/6	10
9-Amino-20($\underline{S}$)-CPT $\underline{9}$	Q04DX02	5(361)	0.6–5	5.97	3/6	10
10-Amino-20(S)-CPT $\underline{10}$[e]	Q04DX02	4.5(565)	2–4.5	>5.99	6/6	*
9-Nitro-20($\underline{S}$)-CPT $\underline{11}$	Q04DX02	10(348)	1.25–20	5.97	5/6	40
9-Amino-10,11-methylenedioxy-20($\underline{S}$)-CPT $\underline{6}$[f]	Q04DX02	1.5(536)	0.3–1.5	5.8	4/6	*
9-Chloro-20($\underline{S}$)-CPT $\underline{16}$	Q04DX02	12(150)	2.37–12.00	0	0/6	*
9-Methyl-20($\underline{S}$)-CPT $\underline{18}$	Q04DX02	8(274)	2.37–8.00	5.6	4/6	12
9-Hydroxy-20($\underline{RS}$)-CPT $\underline{14}$	Q04DX02	20(134)	10–40	*	0/6	*
10-Nitro-20($\underline{RS}$)-CPT $\underline{12}$	Q04DX02	7.25(233)	3.63–15.5	5.97	0/6	31
10-Amino-20($\underline{RS}$)-CPT	Q04DX02	3.75(365)	1.35–3.74	5.97	3/6	6.25
10-Chloro-20($\underline{RS}$)-CPT	Q04DX02	10(280)	5–20	5.97	2/6	40
10,11-Methylenedioxy-20($\underline{RS}$)-CPT $\underline{27}$	Q04DX02	2(325)	2–4	5.97	2/6	8.0

[a]IP implants. [b]Q04DX02 = Drug dosing IP on days 1 and 5. [c]% T/C = (median survival time of treated/median survival time of control animals) × 100. [d]$\log_{10}$ of initial tumor cell population minus $\log_{10}$ of tumor cell population at the end of treatment. [e]100% long-term (day 45) tumor-free survivors. [f]4/6 long-term (day 60) tumor-free survivors. *Data not available.

Table 3 Topoisomerase I inhibition from cleavable complex formation by CPT analogs

Compound	IC-50 (µM)[a]	SE of IC-50[a]
10,11-Methylenedioxy-20(<u>S</u>)-CPT <u>28</u>	0.027	0.005
9-Methyl-20(<u>S</u>)-CPT <u>18</u>	0.038	0.013
9-Amino-10,11-methylenedioxy-20(<u>S</u>)-CPT <u>6</u>	0.048	0.016
9 -Chloro-10,11-methylenedioxy-20(<u>S</u>)-CPT <u>30</u>	0.061	0.019
10,11-Methylenedioxy-20(<u>RS</u>)-CPT <u>27</u>	0.067	0.038
9-Amino-10,11-methylenedioxy-20 (<u>RS</u>)-CPT <u>29</u>	0.076	0.030
9-Chloro-20(<u>S</u>)-CPT <u>16</u>	0.086	0.054
10-Hydroxy- 20(<u>S</u>)-CPT <u>3</u>	0.106	0.031
9-Amino-20(<u>S</u>)-CPT <u>9</u>	0.111	0.024
10-Amino-20(<u>S</u>)-CPT <u>10</u>	0.140	0.022
10-Chloro-20(<u>S</u>)-CPT <u>17</u>	0.141	0.027
10,11-Ethylenedioxy-20(RS)-CPT <u>31</u>	0.468	0.140
10-Nitro-20(<u>S</u>)-CPT <u>13</u>	0.635	0.116
20 (<u>S</u>)-CPT <u>1</u>	0.677	0.215
10,11-Methylenedioxy-20(<u>RS</u>)-CPT, Na⁺Salt <u>36</u>	0.843	0.681
9-Hydroxy-20(<u>S</u>)-CPT <u>15</u>	0.873	0.302
9-Dimethylaminomethyl-10-hydroxy-20(<u>S</u>)-CPT·HCl <u>25</u>	1.110	—
20(RS)-CPT	1.436	0.261
10-Hydroxy-20(<u>S</u>)-CPT, di Na⁺Salt <u>34</u>	3.202	0.603
9,10-Methylenedioxy-20(RS)- CPT <u>32</u>	3.815	0.633
9-Amino-10,11-methylenedioxy-20(<u>S</u>)-CPT, Na⁺Salt <u>33</u>	4.303	2.512
20(<u>S</u>)-CPT, Na⁺Salt <u>2</u>	11.586	5.852
9-Amino-20(<u>RS</u>)-CP·Na⁺Salt <u>35</u>	13.875	5.681
9-Amino-10,11-methylenedioxy-20(<u>R</u>)-CPT	>30	
10,11-Methylenedioxy-20(<u>R</u>)-CPT	>30	
20(<u>R</u>)-CPT	>30	

[a]IC-50 = the minimum drug concentration (µM) that inhibited the cleavable complex formation by 50%.

Active CPT analogs were noted with other substituents in the 9- and 10-positions. For example, the lipophilic 9-chloro-20(<u>S</u>)-CPT (<u>16</u>) and the corresponding 10-chloro-20(<u>RS</u>) analogs have shown activity in inhibition of L-1210 mouse leukemia, and the 9- and 10-chloro-20(<u>S</u>) analogs (<u>16</u>) and (<u>17</u>), respectively, have shown high activity in the T-1 inhibition assay,[18] (cf. Table 3). The 10-chloro-20(<u>RS</u>) analog is also potent *in vivo*, (Table 2). The 9-methyl-20(<u>S</u>) analog (<u>18</u>) has potent activity both in the T-1 and L-1210 *in vivo* assay.[18] Compounds <u>16</u>, <u>17</u>, and <u>18</u> are chloroform soluble, whereas <u>1</u> has low solubility in all solvents except DMSO.

6. Effect of Substitution at C11 and C12

In general, the effect of monosubstitution at C11 and C12 is to lower the activity and/or potency. Of a large number of compounds synthesized with C11 substituents,[15-17] only the 11-cyano-20(<u>RS</u>) (<u>19</u>) and 11-hydroxy-20(<u>RS</u>) (<u>20</u>) analogs exhibited appreciable life prolongation in the murine L1210 leukemia assay, and both compounds had low potency.[15,17] In contrast to the enhancement of activity by amino groups at C9 and C10, the 11-amino-20(<u>RS</u>) analog (<u>21</u>) had low activity, and the 12-amino-20(<u>S</u>) analog (<u>22</u>) was inactive both *in vivo* and *in vitro*.[16,17,20]

7. Effect of Two or More Ring A Substituents

The effects of two or more substituents in the A ring on *in vivo* and/or *in vitro* activity is complex and variable. Moreover, this area still requires considerable study.

a. Analogs Substituted at Both 9 and 10 Positions

A combination of a 10-hydroxy substituent with substituents at C9 results in formation of compounds that are less active than the parent 10-hydroxy-CPT (3) *in vivo* and *in vitro* (T-1 inhibition). Compounds of this type prepared to date are also less active than their mono 9- substituted CPT analogs. Thus, for example, 9-nitro-10-hydroxy-20(S)-CPT (23) is much less active than either 9-nitro-20(S)-CPT (11) or 10-hydroxy-20(S)-CPT (3).[16] Similarly, 9-acetamido-10-hydroxy-20(S)-CPT (24) is less active than the corresponding mono-substituted 10-hydroxy analog (3) or 9-acetamido-20(S)-CPT.[16] 9-Dimethylaminomethyl-10-hydroxy-20(S)-CPT·HCl (25) (Topotecan, SmithKline Beecham, compound currently in clinical trial) is considerably less active than 10-hydroxy-CPT (3) in T-1 inhibition (cf. Table 3, compounds 3, 9, 25, and Section VI entitled "Effect of CPT and Analogs on T-1").

b. Analogs Substituted at Both 10 and 11 Positions

Disubstitution at the 10 and 11 positions, with one notable exception, frequently leads either to inactive or less active compounds. We have previously described the inactivity of 10,11-dimethoxy-20(RS)-CPT (26).[7] The corresponding 10,11-dihydroxy-20(RS)-CPT shows modest activity in L1210 mouse leukemia life prolongation assay, i.e., T/C 157% at a dose of 40 mg/kg. This CPT analog is more active than the dimethoxy analog 26, which is inactive, but it is also much less active than either the corresponding mono-10- or 11-hydroxy analogs of 1.

c. Effects of Substitution of Methylenedioxy and Ethylenedioxy Groups on In Vitro and In Vivo Activity

Substitution of the 10,11-methylenedioxy group in ring A of CPT results in a remarkable enhancement of both *in vivo* (L1210) and *in vitro* activity (T-1 inhibition). Both the 20(RS) (27) and 20(S) (28) analogs are among the most active T-1 inhibition agents[18,20-21] (cf.Table 3). The 20(RS) analog (27) has also shown high activity in the L1210 mouse leukemia assay[16-18,20] and in the inhibition of human xenograft cancer lines in nude mice.[23,24] Recently, we have shown that 9-amino-10,11-methylenedioxy-CPT in either the 20(RS) (29) or 20(S)6 configurations are very active in inhibition of T-1[18] (cf. Table 3). The 20(S) analog (6) is very active and potent in the L1210 mouse leukemia assay (cf.Table 2). The effects of various CPT analogs were studied *in vitro* using B-lymphocytes, which were obtained from patients with B-cell chronic lymphocytic leukemia. B-lymphocytes resistant to chlorambucil and fludarabine, two drugs used in standard treatment, were sensitive to 10,11-20(S)-methylenedioxy-camptothecin (28) and, to an even greater extent, to 9-amino-10,11-methylenedioxy-20(S)-camptothecin (6).[25] Compound 6 had greater cytotoxicity than any other CPT analog tested including the parent 10,11-methylenedioxy analog (28) and was much superior to chlorambucil and fludarabine.[25] The 9-chloro-10,11-methylenedioxy-20(S) analog (30) is also a potent T-1 inhibitor[18] (cf. Table 3).

The 10,11-ethylenedioxy-20(RS) analog (31) is less potent than the corresponding 10,11-methylenedioxy analog (27) but is a more active inhibitor of T-1 than 1[18] (cf. Table 3). 9,10-Methylenedioxy-20(RS)-CPT (32) exhibited considerably reduced T-1 inhibition activity[18] (Table 3). The 10,11-methylenedioxy group is coplanar with ring A and hence does not cause the steric hindrance observed with other 10,11-disubstituted groups. The 10,11-ethylenedioxy moiety is not completely coplanar with ring A, and hence compound 31, because of possible steric interaction, lacks the enhanced activity of the 10,11-methylenedioxy analog. Recent molecular modeling studies have shown that all the

CPT analogs with 10,11-methylenedioxy substituents have much higher max/min values (Kcal mol⁻¹) than CPT and many other CPT analogs (Private communication; A. P. Bowen; Computational Center for Molecular Structure and Design, University of Georgia).

It is conceivable that CPT may bind to an enzyme or enzyme-DNA complex on the face proximal to the C11 and, particularly, the C12 region. Hence, groups substituted in these positions may cause unfavorable steric or stereoelectronic interactions. Substituents at positions C9 and C10 are more distant from this region, and substitution of certain groups at these locations is of less steric consequence. On the other hand, the bulky 9,10-methylenedioxy analog (32), although coplanar to ring A, may bind less well to the T-1-DNA cleavable complex.

8. Water Soluble CPT Analogs

The majority of the water-soluble analogs prepared by us were less potent *in vitro*, T-1 and L1210 *in vivo* (cf. Tables 2, 3, and 5). We have prepared three types of water-soluble analogs (cf. Table 5). Typical examples are (1) sodium salts of the carboxylic acid obtained by hydrolytic cleavage of the ring E lactone,[4,18] (2) 20-glycinate ester-hydrochloride salts,[26] and (3) 9-glycinamido-hydrochloride salts.[18] The objective was to determine if any of these compounds were active per se, or if the glycinate ester and 9-glycinamido hydrochloride salts would be hydrolyzed by esterases and amidases known to be present in human plasma and tissues, or whether facile ring-closure of sodium salts would occur *in vivo*. The results shown in Tables 2 and 4 are typical of a much larger body of data.[18]

a. Sodium Salts

As shown in Table 3, the sodium salts 2, and 33-36 exhibit very weak activity in T-1 inhibition, whereas the corresponding water-insoluble compounds are potent T-1 inhibitors. *In vivo*, compounds 2, 34, and 36 show some activity in L1210 mouse leukemia, albeit of a modest order (cf. Table 5), probably due to some degree of relactonization under physiological conditions. It is evident, however, that extensive relactonization did not occur.

b. 9-Glycinamide Hydrochlorides

We have not studied extensively water-soluble compounds of this type. As shown in Table 5, the 9-glycinamide (37) has modest activity in L1210 mouse leukemia at a relatively high dose by IV administration. T-1 data for this structure was not obtained. Because the parent 9-amino-20(RS)-CPT and the corresponding 20(S) analog 9 are very active in L1210 mouse assays,[16,17] T/C >300% at 3–6 mg/kg, IP, it is evident that significant proportions of 37 were not hydrolyzed under 15 administration conditions.

c. 20-Glycinate Esters

Although much more testing would be required for a definitive conclusion, it would appear that certain water-soluble 20-glycinate esters as exemplified by 38-40 when administered IV at 10–20 mg/kg, afforded substantial life prolongation in the L1210 mouse leukemia assay[18] (cf. Table 5). 1t should be noted that these compounds are 20(RS) analogs. Even more active compounds might be anticipated from the corresponding 20(S) analogs.

9. New Structural Types

Certain new structural types of CPT analogs, which in some cases have been briefly mentioned in earlier sections of this chapter, will be reviewed in terms of biological activity.

Table 4   **Comparison of topoisomerase I inhibition of 20(S), 20 (RS), and 20(R)-CPT compounds**

Compound	IC_{50} (μM)[a]
20(<u>S</u>)-CPT <u>1</u>	0.68
20(<u>RS</u>)-CPT	1.44
20(<u>R</u>)-CPT	>30
9-Amino-20(<u>S</u>)-CPT <u>9</u>	0.11
9-Amino-20(<u>RS</u>)-CPT	0.50
10,11-Methylenedioxy-20(<u>S</u>)-CPT <u>28</u>	0.03
10,11-Methylenedioxy-20(<u>RS</u>)-CPT <u>27</u>	0.08
10,11-Methylenedioxy-20(<u>R</u>)-CPT	>30
9-Amino-10,11-methylenedioxy-20(<u>S</u>)-CPT <u>6</u>	0.05
9-Amino-10,1 1-methylenedioxy-20(<u>RS</u>)-CPT <u>29</u>	0.07
9-Amino-10,11-methylenedioxy-20(<u>R</u>)-CPT	>30

[a]IP implants.

a. Tetracyclic CPT Analog <u>4</u>

In order to determine whether the pentacyclic ring structure of CPT was required for maximal activity, bicyclic ring DE and tricyclic ring CDE compounds with the α-hydroxy-lactone group were prepared and were found to be inactive.[6] A hexacyclic analog was made and found to be of the same order of potency as <u>1</u>.[7] A prediction was made some years ago that the tetracyclic ring de-A analog (<u>4</u>) (cf. Figure 3) might be active.[27] Compound <u>4</u> was prepared with considerable difficulty and was found to be inactive in T-1, IC_{50} =>30μm.[18] It is apparent therefore that the pentacyclic ring structure of CPT is required for activity.

b. Ring D Benzo Analog <u>5</u>

The role of the ring D pyridone moiety has never been clearly understood. The cyclic unsaturated lactam seemed to be relatively unreactive. Synthesis of the ring D benzo CPT analog <u>5</u> was therefore undertaken.[14] Molecular modeling indicated that the shape of the pentacyclic ring D benzo CPT analog was similar to that of <u>1</u>. However, <u>5</u> was found to be almost inactive in the T-1 assay and much less active than <u>1</u> in other cytotoxic assays, such as 9KB and 9PS. Hence, the ring D pyridone moiety is also essential for the *in vitro* and *in vivo* activity of <u>1</u>.

c. Analogs with Variation of C20 Ethyl Substituent

Some years ago, it was noted that the C20 ethyl group could be replaced by allylic groups with no loss of *in vivo* activity.[28] Several new CPT analogs were prepared in which the C20-ethyl group was replaced by CH_3, CH_2CH_2OH, and CH_2CH_2Br, e.g., analogs <u>41</u>, <u>42</u>, and <u>43</u>, respectively.[18] All of the compounds were inactive in T-1 inhibition.

V.   EFFECT OF CPT AND ANALOGS ON TOPOISOMERASE 1 (T-1)

Interest in the potential clinical utilization of CPT (<u>1</u>) or its analogs has been cyclic in intensity. After an initial period of clinical study of the water-soluble sodium salt <u>2</u>, interest lagged due to the inactivity and/or toxicity of this compound.[10-12] Interest greatly increased when it was found that <u>1</u> *interferes with the DNA breakage-reunion reaction*, a biological function exerted by DNA-T-1, by trapping the enzyme-DNA intermediate

Table 5 **L1210 life prolongation[a] by water-soluble CPT analogs**

Compound	Dose Regimen	Route	Highest Active Dose, mg/kg (% T/C)[c]	Dose Range (mg/kg)	KE[d]	Cures	Toxic Dose mg/kg
9-Amino-20-glycinate Ester-20(RS)-CPT·HCI	Q04DX02[b]	IP	10(132)	10	−1.00	0	NT at 10
9-Amino-20 -glycinate Ester-20(RS)-CPT·HCI	Q04HX02[e]	IV	5(168)	2.5–5.0	1.67	1/6	NT at 5
10-Amino-20-glycinate Ester-20(RS)-CPT·HCI	Q04HX02	IV	20(225)	1.25–20	>5.97	0	NT at 20
10,11-Methylenedioxy-20-glycinate Ester-20(RS)-CPT·HCI 39	Q04HX02	IV	10(236)	1.25–20	5.97	3/6	NT at 20
9-Glycinamido-20(RS)-CPT·HCI 37	Q04HX02	IV	20(180)	1.25–20	2.95	0	NT at 20
10,11-Methylenedioxy-20(RS)-CPT Sodium 36	Q04HX02	IV	10(157)	2.85–10	4.79	0	NT at 20
10-Hydroxy-20(S)-CPT Disodium 34	Q04HX02	IV	20(184)	2.5–20	3.24	0	NT at 20

[a]IP implants. [b]Q04DX02 = Drug dosing IP on days 1 and 5. [c]% T/C = (median survival time of treated/median survival time of control animals) × 100. [d]$\log_{10}$ of initial tumor cell population minus $\log_{10}$ of tumor cell population at the end of treatment. [e]Q04HX02 = drug dosing IV, two injections on day 1 and two on day 5.

termed the "cleavable complex".[29,30] The mechanism of inhibition is discussed in detail in Chapter 1.

A. RELATION BETWEEN *IN VIVO* ACTIVITY AND T-1 INHIBITION

There seems to be a reasonable correlation between *in vivo* activity and activity of CPT analogs in the inhibition of T-1 (cf. Tables 2, 3). The relationship is not exact because *in vivo* activity depends not only on the intrinsic structure of the CPT analog but also on many other factors: cell penetration, overall toxicity, plasma binding, solubility, etc. But, in general, inspection of Tables 2 or 3 shows that compounds that have high T-1 inhibition activity also have, for example, excellent life prolongation in the L1210 mouse leukemia assay. Compounds with 20($\underline{S}$) stereochemistry are at least twice as potent as their analogs with the racemic 20($\underline{RS}$) configurations and compounds with the 20($\underline{R}$) configuration are always inactive *in vitro* and *in vivo*, (cf. Tables 3, 4). Some excellent examples of the correlation of *in vivo* activity (L1210) and T-1 inhibition have been shown in a previous study.[20] Thus, the 9-amino-20($\underline{S}$) analog ($\underline{9}$) was potent in both assays, the 11-amino-20($\underline{RS}$) analog ($\underline{21}$) was much less active, and the 12-amino-20($\underline{S}$) analog ($\underline{22}$) was inactive in both assays. A similar relationship was shown for nitro analogs $\underline{11}$ and $\underline{12}$, the nitro analog $\underline{11}$ being the more active *in vivo* (cf. Table 2).[16,17,20] The corresponding 11- and 12-nitro analogs are progressively less active. The high potency in assays of both the 20($\underline{RS}$)- and 20($\underline{S}$)-10,11-methylenedioxy analogs $\underline{27}$ and $\underline{28}$ is demonstrated by comparison of data in Tables 2 and 3.[20,21]

1. Effect of Prodrugs

The correlations of *in vivo* assays and T-1 inhibition activities are so good that, in general, initial assessment of the potential *in vivo* activity of a new CPT analog can be carried out rapidly by use of the T-1 inhibition assay (cf. Tables 2 and 3).[20] The case of prodrugs which might be weakly active in T-1 inhibition but which can be bioactively converted to active compounds are exceptions. This is the case with the Japanese compound CPT 11, a water-soluble derivative of 7-ethyl-10-hydroxy-20($\underline{S}$)-CPT which is converted *in vivo* to the active 7-ethyl-10-hydroxy compound.[31,32]

B. RELATIONSHIPS BETWEEN STRUCTURE OF CAMPTOTHECIN AND ANALOGS AND T-1 INHIBITION

As a consequence of the successful resolution of the ($\underline{RS}$) tricyclic synthon, the chiral ($\underline{S}$) and ($\underline{R}$) synthons are now readily available (cf. Figure 3).[18] Friedlander reactions of the chiral tricyclic synthons with appropriately substituted ortho-aminobenzaldehydes have yielded for the first time chiral 20($\underline{S}$) and 20($\underline{R}$)-CPT analogs.[18] Table 3 presents T-1 inhibition IC_{50} values for a number of 20($\underline{S}$) and a few 20($\underline{RS}$) and 20($\underline{R}$) analogs substituted for the most part in the 9, 10, or 10,11- positions. The T-1 inhibition data are compared directly in Table 4 for selected CPT analogs.

The CPT analogs are listed in Table 3 in order of decreasing potency against purified T-1 (as assessed by formation of the cleavable complex), and the discussion will relate in this case to the IC_{50} potency data. Four distinct classes of potency can be more or less arbitrarily assigned: Class 1, compounds with IC_{50} values between 0.01 and 0.10 µM; Class 2, compounds with values between 0.1–1.0 µM; Class 3, compounds with values between 1.0–10.0 µM; and Class 4, compounds with values >10.0 µM.

Data in Table 4 shows that the 20($\underline{S}$) form of a particular CPT analog is always much more potent than the 20($\underline{R}$) form and is approximately twice as potent as the 20($\underline{RS}$) form (range 1.5–4.0 fold).

1. Water-Insoluble CPT Analogs

The compounds with maximal IC_{50} values in general are water-insoluble 20($\underline{S}$) and 20($\underline{RS}$) analogs substituted in the 9 or 10 position. CPT analogs 9-amino ($\underline{9}$), 10-hydroxy ($\underline{3}$), 9-chloro-10,11-methylenedioxy ($\underline{30}$), or 9-methyl ($\underline{18}$) show in general high T-1 inhibition activity. The relatively low activity of 9-hydroxy-20($\underline{S}$)-CPT ($\underline{15}$) is an exception. The presence of a 10,11-methylenedioxy substituent, for example, in analogs $\underline{27}$ and $\underline{28}$, greatly enhances the basic CPT activity, either when present singly or when 9-amino or 9-chloro substitutents are also present as in analogs $\underline{6}$ or $\underline{30}$. Planarity of the substituents in ring A appears crucial for enhancing the biological activity of the various CPT analogs. For example, the 10,11-ethylenedioxy-20($\underline{RS}$) analog ($\underline{31}$), which is less planar, is only about one-seventh as potent in T-1 inhibition as the corresponding 10,11-methylenedioxy-20($\underline{RS}$) analog ($\underline{27}$). Moreover, the location of the planar substituent in ring A also appears to be crucial for activity. Thus the planar analog, 9,10-ethylenedioxy-20($\underline{RS}$)-CPT ($\underline{32}$) has only one-fiftieth the activity of $\underline{27}$.

2. Water-Soluble Analogs

Water-soluble analogs which cannot undergo bioactive transformation in the T-1 assay or which interact poorly with the DNA-T-1 cleavable complex show poor-to-modest activity in T-1 inhibition. Compare in Table 3, for example, $\underline{27}$ with the corresponding sodium salt $\underline{36}$, and 10-hydroxy-20($\underline{S}$)-CPT ($\underline{3}$) with the corresponding water-soluble analog $\underline{34}$.

As shown in Tables 3 and 4, all the 20($\underline{R}$) analogs are essentially inactive in T-1 inhibition. 20($\underline{R}$)-CPT has been shown to be inactive also in 9KB cytotoxicity and in the *in vivo* L1210 mouse leukemia assay.[19,20]

VI.   CONCLUSIONS

A. DRUGS CURRENTLY IN CLINICAL TRIAL

At present,CPT ($\underline{1}$) and three CPT analogs, 9-amino-20($\underline{S}$)-CPT ($\underline{9}$), 9-dimethylaminomethyl-10-hydroxy-20($\underline{S}$)-CPT·HCl (Topotecan ($\underline{25}$)), and CPT 11, a water-soluble analog of 7-ethyl-10-hydroxy-20($\underline{S}$)-CPT, are in clinical trial. Water-insoluble $\underline{1}$, administered orally, has recently entered Phase II clinical trial (Chapter 4). As a consequence of studies which showed that water-insoluble $\underline{9}$ exhibited high *in vivo* antitumor activity in the L1210 assay,[12,16,17] remarkable activity in human xenograft colorectal tumors[23] in conjunction with high T-1 inhibition,[20] and because of the development of a parenteral infusion procedure by the National Cancer Institute, $\underline{9}$ is now receiving Phase I clinical trial. Water-soluble drugs Topotecan and CPT-11 have been in clinical trial for several years, and some results are now available. Clinical trials of CPT, CPT-11, and Topotecan are discussed in detail in other chapters.

Several other CPT analogs may eventually receive consideration for clinical trial. These include the 10-amino analog $\underline{10}$ and the 9-amino-10,11-methylenedioxy analog $\underline{6}$, both highly active in L1210 mouse leukemia assay (cf. Table 2). Compound $\underline{6}$ has recently been shown to have considerable cytotoxicity toward B-cell chronic lymphocytic leukemia (CLL) cells with activity much greater than chlorambucil, a drug currently in clinical use for CLL patients, or other CPT analogs.[25]

Recently, two new water-soluble CPT analogs with a water-solubilizing moiety, N-methylpiperazinomethyl in ring B at C7 and, respectively, 10,11-methylenedioxy or 10,11-ethylenedioxy groups in ring A have been reported. The compounds exhibited potent antitumor activity *in vivo* in xenograft models of human colon, breast, prostate, and lung cancer. Entry into clinical trial is expected by 1994.

ACKNOWLEDGMENTS

We thank Dr. Jeffrey Besterman, Glaxo, Inc., for T-1 inhibition data. Many of the compounds reported in this chapter have been the result of skilled experimental research by Drs. Allan Nicholas and Govindarajan Manikumar. The research reported in this chapter has been supported by NIH-NCI CA-38996-01-06 and CA50529.

REFERENCES

1. **Perdue, R. E., Jr., Smith, R. L., Wall, M. E., Hartwell, J. L., and Abbott, B. J.,** *Camptotheca acuminata* Decaisne (Nyssaceae). Source of camptothecin, an antileukemic alkaloid, U.S. Department of Agriculture, *Agric. Res. Serv. Tech. Bull.,* No. 1415, 1 (1970).
2. **Wall, M. E.,** Discovery of camptothecin and taxol, in *Chronicles of Drug Discovery,* Vol. 3, Lednicer, D., Ed., American Chemical Society, Washington, D. C., 1993, in press.
3. **Geran, R. I., Greenberg, N. H., MacDonald, M. M., Schumacher, A. M., and Abbott, B.J.,** Protocols for screening chemical agents and natural products against animal tumors and other biological systems, 3rd ed., *Cancer Chemotherapy Repts.,* 3, 1, 1972.
4. **Wall, M. E., Wani, M. C., Cook, C. E., Palmer, K. H., McPhail, A. T., and Sim, G. A.,** Plant antitumor agents. 1. The isolation and structure of camptothecin: a novel alkaloidal leukemia and tumor inhibitor from *Camptotheca acuminata, J. Am. Chem. Soc.,* 88, 3888, 1966.
5. **Wani, M. C. and Wall, M. E.,** Plant antitumor agents. 2. The structure of two new alkaloids from *Camptotheca acuminata, J. Org. Chem.,* 34, 1364, 1969.
6. **Wall, M. E.,** Plant antitumor agents. 5. Alkaloids with antitumor activity, *Symposiumsberichtes,* Mothes, K., Schreiber, K., and Schutte, H. R., Eds., Akademie-Verlag, Berlin, 1969, 77.
7. **Wani, M. C., Ronman, P. E., Lindley, J. T., and Wall, M. E.,** Plant antitumor agents. 18. Synthesis and biological activity of camptothecin analogs, *J. Med. Chem.,* 23, 554, 1980.
8. **Gottlieb, J. A., Guarino, A. M., Call, J. B., Oliverio, V. T., and Block, J. B.,** Preliminary pharmacologic and clinical evaluation of camptothecin sodium, *Cancer Chemother. Rep.,* 54, 461, 1970.
9. **Muggia, F. M., Creaven, P. J., Jansen, H. A., Cohen, M. H., and Selawry, O. S.,** Phase I clinical trial of weekly and daily schedules of camptothecin sodium: correlation with preclinical studies, *Cancer Chemother. Rep.,* 56, 515, 1972.
10. **Moertel, C. G., Schutt, A. J., Reitemeier, R. J., and Hahn, R. G.,** Phase II study of camptothecin in the treatment of advanced gastrointestical cancer, *Cancer Chemother. Rep.,* 56, 95, 1972.
11. **Xu, B.,** Clinical studies with camptothecin sodium, in *U.S./China Pharmacology Symposium,* Burns, J. J. and Tsuchiatani, P. J., Eds., National Academy of Sciences, Washington, D. C., 1980, 156.
12. **Wall, M. E. and Wani, M. C.,** Chemistry and antitumor activity of camptothecins, in *DNA Topoisomerases in Cancer,* Potmesil, M. and Kohn, K. W., Eds., Oxford University Press, New York, 1991, 93.
13. **Cai, J. C. and Hutchinson, C. R.,** Camptothecin, in *Alkaloids,* Vol. 21, Brossi, A., Ed., Academic Press, New York, 1983, chap. 4.
14. **Nicholas, A. W., Wani, M. C., Manikumar, G., Wall, M. E., Kohn, K. W., and Pommier, Y.,** Plant antitumor agents. 29. Synthesis and biological activity of ring D and ring E modified analogs of camptothecin, *J. Med. Chem.,* 33, 972, 1990.

15. **Wall, M. E., Wani, M. C., Natschke, S. M., and Nicholas, A. W.,** Plant antitumor agents.22. Isolation of 11-hydroxycamptothecin from *Camptotheca acuminata* decne: Total synthesis and biological activity, *J. Med. Chem.*, 29, 1553, 1986.

16. **Wani, M. C., Nicholas, A. W., and Wall, M. E.,** Plant antitumor agents. 23. Synthesis and antileukemic activity of camptothecin analogues, *J. Med. Chem.*, 29, 2358, 1986.

17. **Wani, M. C., Nicholas, A. W., Manikumar, G., and Wall, M. E.,** Plant antitumor agents. 25. Total synthesis and antileukemic activity of ring A-substituted camptothecin analogs, structure activity, *J. Med. Chem.*, 30, 1774, 1987.

18. **Wall, M. E., Wani, M. C., Nicholas, A. W., Manikumar, G., Tele, C., Moore, L., Truesdale, A., Leitner, P., and Besterman, J. M.,** Plant antitumor agents. 30. Synthesis and structure activity of novel camptothecin analogs, *J. Med. Chem.*, 1993, in press.

19. **Wani, M. C., Nicholas, A. W., and Wall, M. E.,** Plant Antitumor Agents. 28. Resolution of a key tricyclic synthon, 5′($\underline{RS}$)-1,5-dioxo-(5′-ethyl-5′hydroxy-2′$\underline{H}$, 5′$\underline{H}$, 6′$\underline{H}$-6-oxopyrano)[3′,4′-$\underline{f}$]^{6,8}-tetrahydroindolizine: total synthesis and antitumor activity of 20($\underline{S}$)- and 20($\underline{R}$)-camptothecin, *J. Med. Chem.*, 30, 2317, 1987.

20. **Jaxel, C., Kohn, K. W., Wani, M. C., and Wall, M. E.,** Structure activity study of the actions of camptothecin derivatives on mammalian topoisomerase I, evidence for a specific receptor site and for a relation to antitumor activity, *Cancer Res.*, 49, 1465, 1989.

21. **Hsiang, Y.-H., Liu, L. F., Wall, M. E., Wani, M. C., Kirschenbaum, S., Silber, R., and Potmesil, M.,** DNA topoisomerase I-mediated DNA cleavage and cytotoxicity of camptothecin analogs, *Cancer Res.*, 49, 4385, 1989.

22. **Wall, M. E. and Wani, M. C.,** Antitumor and topoisomerase I, inhibition activity of camptothecin and analogs, in *Economic and Medicinal Plant Research*, Vol. 5, Wagner, H., Hekino, H., and Farnsworth, N. R., Eds., Academic Press, New York, 1991, chap. 5.

23. **Giovanella, B. C., Stehlin, J. S., Wall, M. E., Wani, M. C., Nicholas, A. W., Liu, L. F., Silber, R., and Potmesil, M.,** Highly effective DNA topoisomerase I-targeted chemotherapy of human colon cancer in xenografts, *Science*, 246, 1046, 1989.

24. **Potmesil, M., Giovanella, B. C., Liu, L. F., Wall, M. E., Silber, R., Stehlin, J. S., Hsiang, Y.-H, and Wani, M. C.,** Preclinical studies of DNA topoisomerase I-targeted 9-amino and 10,11-methylenedioxy camptothecins, in *DNA Topoisomerases in Cancer*, Potmesil, M. and Kohn, K. W., Eds., Oxford University Press, New York, 1991, 299.

25. **Costin, D., Potmesil, M., Morse, L., Mani, M., Canellakis, Z. W., and Silber, R.,** Sensitivity of chronic leukemia B lymphocytes to camptothecin analogs, in *Abstracts of the Fourth Conference on DNA Topoisomerases in Therapy*, No. 62, New York, 1992, 53.

26. **Vishnuvajjala, B. R., Cradock, J. C., and Garzon-Aburbek, A.,** Water-soluble camptothecin prodrugs, *Pharm. Res.*, 3, 22S.

27. **Flurry, Jr., R. L. and Howland, J. C.,** A molecular orbital study of camptothecin and some of its substructures, in *Abstracts of Papers, 162nd Meeting of the American Chemical Society*, Washington, D.C., 1971, 30.

28. **Sugasawa, T., Toyoda, T., Uchida, J., and Yamaguchi, K.,** Experiments on the synthesis of dl-camptothecin. 4. Synthesis and antileukemic activity of dl-camptothecin analogues, *J. Med. Chem.*, 19, 675, 1976.

29. **Hsiang, Y.-H., Hertzberg, R., Hecht, S., and Liu, L. F.,** Camptothecin-induced protein-linked DNA breaks via mammalian DNA topoisomerase I, *J. Biol. Chem.*, 260, 14873, 1985.

30. **Hsiang, Y.-H. and Liu, L. F.,** Identification of mammalian DNA topoisomerase I as an intracellular target of the anticancer drug camptothecin, *Cancer Res.*, 48, 1722, 1988.

31. **Kingsbury, W. D., Boehm, J. C., Dalia, R. J., Holden, K. G., Hecht, S. M., Gallagher, G., Caranea, M. J., McCabe, F. L., Faucette, C. F., Johnson, R. K., and Herzberg, R. P.,** Synthesis of water-soluble (aminoalkyl) camptothecin analogs: inhibition of topoisomerase I and antitumor activity, *J. Med. Chem.*, 34, 98, 1991.

32. **Sawada, S., Okayima, S., Aiyama, R., Ken-ichiro, N., Furuta, T., Yokokura, T., Sugino, E., Yamaguchi, K., and Miyasaka, T.,** Synthesis and antitumor activity of 20($\underline{S}$)-camptothecin derivatives: carbamate-linked, water-soluble derivatives of 7-Ethyl-10-hydroxycamptothecin, *Chem. Pharm. Bull.*, 39, 1446, 1991.

Chapter 3

Twenty Years Later: Review of Clinical Trials with Camptothecin Sodium (NSC-100880)

Franco Muggia

CONTENTS

I. INTRODUCTION

Following its isolation from the stemwood of *Camptotheca acuminata*, and demonstration of camptothecin's activity against L1210 murine leukemia and the rat Walker carcinosarcoma,[1] the National Cancer Institute (NCI) proceeded to formulate the compound for clinical trial as the water-soluble sodium salt (NSC-100880). Preclinical studies had indicated several distinct biochemical and biological properties: (1) potent inhibition of DNA and RNA synthesis in leukemic cells and in normal lymphocyte cultures,[2-5] (2) effects on RNA synthesis lagging behind DNA synthesis and initially reversible,[3-5] (3) cytotoxicity to normal lymphocytes only if undergoing cell division,[6] and (4) optimal activity against L1210 leukemia on a day 1, 5, and 9 dosing schedule. Clinical studies, coupled with evaluation of its pharmacology, were therefore begun at the NCI's Baltimore Cancer Research Center facility by the late Jeffrey Gottlieb working in close collaboration with Anthony Guarino and Vincent Oliverio of the Laboratory of Chemical Pharmacology, Chemotherapy Program, NCI.

Results of this initial study were published in 1970,[7] and internal communications had already prompted a second Phase I study to be initiated at the then recently established NCI-Washington Veterans Administration (VA) unit. This study, conducted by this author as senior investigator, was to explore tolerance of a weekly and subsequently of daily × 5 schedules. While this second study was ongoing during 1970, publicity in the lay press about activity seen against metastatic adenocarcinomas of enteric origin in several patients, prompted Phase II studies to be initiated at the Mayo Clinic (under the direction of Charles Moertel), as well as extensive planting of the trees from which the drug was isolated in property owned by the U.S. Department of Agriculture around Chico, California. A bright future was anticipated for this drug, and this last maneuver sought to avoid sole reliance on its extraction from trees growing in mainland China, which were off limits to U.S. interests.

The clinical results of these original studies are here reviewed,[7-9] as well as an additional subsequent Phase II study in malignant melanoma conducted by Gottlieb and Luce at MD Anderson.[10] These studies represent the totality of clinical experience with camptothecin sodium (CS). Other publications dealing with drug pharmacology also appeared shortly thereafter.[7,11-16] However, after Moertel's presentation at the American Association for Cancer Research (AACR) in May 1971 on the results of his Phase II study, interest in developing this drug further declined rapidly. Toxic manifestations in this Phase II study overshadowed new information from mechanistic studies by Susan Horwitz and colleagues at Albert Einstein's pharmacology department that demonstrated antiviral and DNA cleaving properties of the drug.[17-21] These investigators confirmed earlier observation by Wall[22] that the lactone ring was essential for camptothecin's activity, and that the sodium salt with the open carboxylic configuration only became active in an acid pH when the reaction's equilibrium shifted to favor the closed lactone form in the E ring of camptothecin.[23-24] Also overshadowed were preclinical studies by Ira Kline and Abraham Goldin demonstrating synergistic effects of ICRF-159 and camptothecin sodium against intraperitoneal L1210 leukemia. Results from these experiments appear as a table in a book chapter.[25] The discussion to follow will interpret this early clinical and preclinical data with our current perspective and conclude with comments on their possible relevance to clinical investigations with the new camptothecin derivatives, as well as other topoisomerase I and II inhibitors.

II. RESULTS AND DISCUSSION

Prior to human trials with CS, toxicology was carried out in four animal species (information available for NCI protocol design, 1969–1970). In the mouse, the optimal results in L1210 leukemic bearing mice were obtained with a dose of 40 mg/kg given on days 1, 5, 9 which was associated with seven of eight normal mice surviving (i.e., approximately the LD_{10}). A single dose of 80 mg/kg was well tolerated, whereas 4 mg/kg days 1–9 (total dose 36 mg/kg) again resulted in one lethal event in eight normal mice.[8] Single doses of CS in rats indicated an LD_{10} between 600 and 800 mg/m^2 and an LD_{50} of 1000 mg/m^2; enterocolitis contributed to deaths. The dog proved as tolerant to single drug doses as the rat, and other schedules showed clear schedule dependency. On a weekly $\times$ 6 schedule, up to 400 mg/m^2 per week was tolerated with diarrhea, leukopenia, and thrombocytopenia being noted; whereas 200 mg/m^2/week was nontoxic. On a daily schedule, 40 mg/m^2/day $\times$ 6 was lethal in two of two animals, and 20 mg/m^2/d $\times$ 9 and 15 mg/m^2/d $\times$ 14 were lethal in one of two animals. Monkeys showed similar lethality when dosed at 40 mg/m^2/d $\times$ 6 and at 15 mg/m^2 $\times$ 14. Deaths were due to both hemorrhagic enterocolitis and leukopenia. On the other hand, 7 mg/m^2/d $\times$ 14 was not obviously toxic to the dog. These results indicate that single doses are equally well tolerated by the rat and the dog, that dogs and monkeys show analogous intolerance to much lower daily doses, and that the mouse is somewhat more sensitive to both single doses and repeated daily $\times$ 9 doses (LD_{10} approximately 240 mg/m^2 and 12 mg/m^2, respectively).

The initial clinical study of CS[7] consisted of a dose-escalating trial of single intravenous push doses beginning at 0.5 mg/kg (approximately 15 mg/m^2) and escalating to a maximum of 10 mg/kg (350 mg/m^2). Doses were given every two to four weeks to 16 patients with adult solid tumors, who received 35 courses. Two additional patients, one of whom had acute myelogenous leukemia, received 2 to 2.5 mg/kg every three days for five doses. Dose-limiting myelosuppression was encountered, consisting primarily of thrombocytopenia and leukopenia at the highest dose levels. Other toxicities reported were alopecia, hemorrhagic cystitis, and gastrointestinal symptoms. A dose of 5 to 7.5 mg/kg every two weeks was recommended for further study, and four partial responses (PRs), albeit brief (median 2+ months), were reported among ten patients with carcinoma of gastrointestinal origin and one PR in a melanoma lymph node. Evidence of antitumor activity was noted in six other patients. Although this enthusiastic assessment of activity in a Phase I study is unusual, it is even more noteworthy that Gottlieb preferentially selected patients with bowel cancer for study based on animal toxicology indicating hemorrhagic colitis as one of its prominent manifestations. Subsequent preclinical studies with camptothecin and derivatives (Chapter 3) and clinical experience with CPT-11 (Chapters 6 to 10) vindicate the validity of these original observations.

The weekly schedule was explored at the NCI-VA Medical Oncology Service to follow up on L1210 data which indicated optimal activity on an intermittent days 1, 5, 9 schedule. The starting dose was 67 mg/m^2, which represented about one half of the recommended single dose reported in the above trial by Gottlieb. At this dose, mild leukopenia (WBC median 3.5, range of 2.6–4.4 $\times$ 10^3 mm^3) and thrombocytopenia (platelet count median 126, range of 97–327 $\times$ 10^3/mm^3) were observed in four patients after a median of 2, and a range of 1 to 3 weekly doses. An additional 11 patients received 17 courses at 44, 30, and 20 mg/m^2/w in a deescalation trial for the unusual purpose of establishing a minimally toxic weekly dose. Reticulocytopenia followed by anemia was universal and most pronounced at the highest dose. Unfortunately, cystitis occurred in four patients at the lower doses; and gastrointestinal toxicities such as nausea and vomiting in two patients and diarrhea in one patient at the highest dose. Rebound reticulocytosis and thrombocytosis were documented in some patients. There were two responses out of a total of 15 patients treated (ten evaluable for response): one in a patient presenting with Stage IV lung adenocarcinoma with a PR in an axillary lymph node lasting two months receiving 67 mg/m^2/w and one complete response (CR) with no subsequent relapse in a patient with a presumed Stage I gastric cancer with medical contraindications for surgery receiving 44 mg/m^2/w.[8] This latter patient experienced severe urethritis, cystitis, and total alopecia after two doses, only to reexperience these symptoms when another dose was given several weeks later.

The same trial was extended to evaluate a daily $\times$ 5 schedule in order to provide a suitable dose for Phase II studies to be used at the Mayo Clinic that was to explore both high-intermittent doses and this new schedule in patients with gastrointestinal cancer, where interest remained high. Because of the preclinical data cited above, the trial began at a starting dose of 0.3 mg/m^2/d $\times$ 5 in cohorts of three patients/level. Seven dose escalations were carried out below a cumulative 5-day dose of 43 mg/m^2 without any consistent toxicities being seen; cystitis was noted in one patient. Toxicities similar to those of the weekly schedule were observed at cumulative 5-day doses of 56, 75, and 100 mg/m^2. Six courses of this last dose were given, resulting in a median white cell nadir of 2.9 $\times$ 10^3/mm^3 on day 1. One course given at 120 mg/m^2 resulted in a granulocyte nadir of 1400/.1 cumm. Cystitis occurred in 3 of 17 patients receiving these 5-day courses. No objective antitumor responses were documented.[8] When compared to the preclinical toxicology, the equivalent dose tolerance of 5-day courses relative to the weekly or single intermittent courses was unexpected.

As already noted, premature press releases on the activity of CS against gastrointestinal cancer prompted initiation of Phase II trials at the Mayo Clinic under the direction of Charles Moertel.[9] The initial trial explored single intermittent dosing in patients with a variety of gastrointestinal tumors, predominantly colon, some of whom had experienced prior therapies. The initial dose of 180 mg/m^2 proved too toxic and was deescalated to 110 mg/m^2 and subsequently to 90 mg/m^2 every three weeks. Toxicities were similar to those in the Phase I study, but severe nausea and vomiting and hematologic toxicities were more prominent at the highest doses. One drug-related death was recorded in a patient with hydronephrosis, among 34 patients entered. Toxicities are shown in Table 1, in comparison with the toxicities experienced by 27 patients subsequently entered on a 5-day course study. Two objective PRs among 30 patients with colon cancer occurred with this single intermittent dosing schedule.

Table 1   Toxicities of camptothecin sodium in phase II*

Toxicity		Percent Toxicities	
		Single Treatment (N = 34)	5-day Treatment (N = 27)
Vomiting		41	41
Diarrhea		21	37
Stomatitis		12	11
Cystitis		24	48**
Dermatitis		—	7
Alopecia		71	87
Leukopenia	<4000	47	35
	<2000	22	19
Thrombopenia	<1000,m000)	13	23
	<50,000	7	12
Anemia	(dec >2 gm Hb)	15	39**
Drug-related deaths		1	2

*Modified from Reference 9. **p<0.05.

A second trial at the Mayo Clinic explored 5-day courses in 27 patients with gastrointestinal cancer who received 11 to 22 mg/m^2/d of CS in accordance to results from the previously described Phase I study. This schedule proved more toxic than the intermittent schedule in two respects: anemia and cystitis (Table 1). No responses were seen in this toxic schedule, leading the authors to conclude that "Camptothecin is a drug of protean and unpredictable toxicity that has no clinical value in the management of gastrointestinal cancer".[9] At the May 1971 AACR presentation in Chicago, Moertel concluded with a picture of the new crop of *Camptotheca acuminata* trees in California and the comment that "the tree is not pretty, and the roots are not even edible".[26]

Gottlieb, by this time at the MD Anderson Hospital, launched one additional attempt to prove the value of CS. Because of a minor response in a patient with melanoma in his original trial, he designed a Phase II study on an every two week schedule, starting at 90 mg/m^2 with built-in dose escalations according to individual tolerance. Several patients were escalated, one as far up as 360 mg/m^2. Fifteen patients were treated, but no responses were observed.[10] Table 2 summarizes this entire clinical experience with CS taking place between 1969 and 1972.

Pharmacologic studies had been performed during Gottlieb's original Phase I study. Using a fluorometric assay,[11] the authors reported a high degree of protein binding of CS so that fluorescence was still detectable six days later. Urinary excretion accounted for only 17.4% of unmetabolized drug in 48h.[6] The biliary route of excretion for the drug was documented by Guarino and Call.[14] Utilizing a similar fluorometric assay, Creaven et al. studied patients entered in our NCI-VA 5-day course study.[16] Interpatient variation in peak plasma levels was considerable, ranging between 0.25 and 1.5 mcg/ml after 11 to 25 mg/m^2/d. There was a tendency for increasing peak levels on consecutive days, but some patients showed a stepwise decline after onset of hydration, which correlated with increased renal clearance of the drug.[15] The equilibrium between the lactone (closed) and carboxylic (open) forms was not known at the time.

III.   CONCLUSION

The history of early trials with CS has some interest in reminding us about pitfalls in clinical drug development, and the changes in drug evaluation that have taken place in the

Table 2 **Clinical experience with camptothecin sodium (1969–1972)**

First Author	Phase	Schedule	No. Patients	Doses Range mg/m^2/Course	Ref.
Gottlieb	I	q2w	18	15–350	7
Muggia	I	qw	15	20–67	8
		daily × 5	18	1.5–120	
Moertel	II	q3w	34	90–180	9
	(G.I)	daily × 5	27	55–110	
Gottlieb	II	q2w	15	90–360	10
	(melanoma)				

past 20 years, which we now take for granted (e.g., the need to study a homogeneous population in Phase II, to identify good risk versus poor risk patients, etc.). However, this chapter has reviewed in depth early findings because they may also hold lessons for the clinical development of currently introduced camptothecin derivatives. Among them are the following:

A. CONSIDERATIONS IN SCHEDULING

This issue is not entirely dependent on pharmacokinetics. What needs to be considered is differential cytotoxicity between normal target tissues (gastrointestinal tract, marrow) and the tumor which may be supported by higher Topl levels in malignant as opposed to normal tissues. In addition, in developing dose schedules for Phase II testing, one needs to consider interpatient variability in dose-limiting toxicities (perhaps reflecting pharmacokinetics). The clinical experience with CS (consistent with preclinical L1210 data and with xenograft data with the current derivatives; see Chapter 4) suggests intermittent scheduling has superior antitumor activity and tolerance. Moreover, up to a four-fold escalation in dose was safely accomplished when individual patients were dose-escalated every two weeks.

B. PHARMACOKINETIC CONSIDERATIONS

Toxicity to normal target tissues is likely to be related in part to pharmacokinetic considerations, which in turn relate to the equilibrium between open (inactive) and closed (active) forms of the E ring. The extent of protein binding is another major determinant of potency in relation to dose and renal clearances. Finally, lipophilicity constitutes yet another variable. Topotecan is a potent drug that is less protein bound; the lactone has a slower clearance than the open form, with a beta half-life following 24 h infusions of up to 7.5 mg/m^2 in children of approximately 3h.[27] Urinary recovery after 24 h infusions ranged between 87 and 99%. The dose-limiting toxicity after 24 h infusions is granulocytopenia with or without thrombocytopenia. CPT-11, on the other hand, is a lipophilic prodrug of the more potent SN-38. It has shown activity against colorectal cancer[28] and other tumors in doses of 100 mg/m^2 every week or 150 mg/m^2 every two weeks; pharmacokinetics of drug and prodrug show considerable interpatient variability.[29] Hematologic toxicities are similar to camptothecin and topotecan, but diarrhea is prominent in high-dose intermittent schedules. The 9-amino derivative of camptothecin has entered clinical trials under NCI sponsorship: comparative pharmacokinetics and toxicology events will be of interest. Correlations between drug exposure to the lactone form and toxicities such as myelosuppression should prove helpful in making toxicity more predictable in relation to pharmacokinetic parameters. However, similar AUC correlations would be needed with antitumor effects in order to predict optimal scheduling.

C. FUTURE RESEARCH TARGETS

As we view the early experience with CS 20 years later, it lends support to the initial exploration of this drug in gastrointestinal cancer as a preferred disease target, which has been further supported by substantial preclinical and clinical leads (covered in other chapters). The short responses observed cause concern over development of drug resistance, which is shared by current studies. Laboratory findings are providing guidance into issues related to drug resistance, collateral sensitivity to other topoisomerase-mediated drugs, and the rational development of drug combinations. In this respect, the empirical finding of synergy between ICRF-159, a *bis*(2,6-dioxopiperazine), and CS in L1210 leukemia may be relevant. *Bis*(2,6-dioxopiperazines) inhibit DNA topoisomerase II activity without forming cleavable complexes.[30,31] Hopefully, the early clinical and preclinical experience with CS will shed some light on the clinical development of the recently introduced camptothecins when given alone. In addition, subject of much current study are EORTC and NCI sponsored trials pursuing combination of these drugs with Taxol, Taxotere, cisplatin, or 5FU.

ACKNOWLEDGMENTS

The author is indebted to Patrick Creaven, Susan Horwitz, John Nitiss, and Dan Von Hoff for helpful comments during preparation of this chapter. Dianne Moody provided invaluable assistance in preparation of the finished manuscript. Former co-workers and patients of two decades ago at the NCI and the NCI-VA are gratefully remembered for their selfless participation.

REFERENCES

1. **Wall, M. E., Wani, M. C., Cook, C. E., Palmer, K. H., McPhail, A. T., and Sim, G. A.,** Plant antitumor agents. 1. The isolation and structure of camptothecin, a novel alkaloidal leukemia and tumor inhibitor from *Camptotheca acuminata. J. Am. Chem. Soc.* 83:3888-3890, 1966.

2. **Venditti, J. M. and Abbott, B. J.,** Studies of oncolytic agents from natural sources. Correlations of activity against animal tumors and clinical effectiveness. *Lloydia.* 30:332-348, 1967.

3. **Kessel, D.,** Effects of camptothecin on RNA synthesis in leukemia L1210 cells. *Biochem. Biophys. Acta.* 246:225-232, 1971.

4. **Hacker, B., Keude, A. S., and Hall, T. S.,** Effects of camptothecin and its chemical intermediates upon nucleic acid biosynthesis in L1210 mouse leukemia cells. *Fed. Proc.* 30:2409, 1971.

5. **Kahn, H. E., Jr., Snyder, A. L., and Kohn, K. W.,** Effects of chemotherapeutic agents on RNA synthesis in L1210 cells. *Proc. Am. Assoc. Cancer Res.* 12:59, 1971.

6. **Gallo, R. C., Whang-Peng, J., and Adamson, R. H.,** Studies on the antitumor activity, mechanism of action, and cell cycle effects of camptothecin. *J. Natl. Cancer Inst.* 46:789-795, 1971.

7. **Gottlieb, J. A., Guarino, A. M., Call, J. B., Oliverio, V. T., and Block, J. B.,** Preliminary pharmacologic and clinical evaluation of camptothecin sodium (NSC-100880). *Cancer Chemother. Rep.* 54:461-479, 1970.

8. **Muggia, F. M., Creaven, P. J., Hansen, H. H., Cohen, M. H., and Selawry, O. S.,** Phase I clinical trial of weekly and daily oral treatment with camptothecin sodium (NSC-100880): correlation with preclinical studies. *Cancer Chemother. Rep.* 56:515-521, 1972.

9. **Moertel, C. G., Schutt, A. J., Reitemeier, R. J., and Hahn, R. G.,** Phase II sudy of camptothecin (NSC-100880) in the treatment of advanced gastrointestinal cancer. *Cancer Chemother. Rep.* 56:95-101, 1972.

10. **Gottlieb, J. A. and Luce, J. K.,** Treatment of malignant lymphoma with camptothecin (NSC-100880). *Cancer Chemother. Rep.* 56:103-105, 1972.

11. **Hart, L. G., Call, J. B., and Oliverio, V. T.,** A fluorimetric method for determination of camptothecin in plasma and urine. *Cancer Chemother. Rep.* 53:211-214, 1969.

12. **Guarino, A. M. and Call, J. B.,** Biliary excretion of sodium camptothecin, an antitumor alkaloid with a novel ring system. *Fed. Proc.* 29:543, 1970.

13. **Sieber, S. M., Mead, J. A. R., and Adamson, R. H.,** Pharmacology of antitumor agents from higher plants. *Cancer Treat. Rep.* 60:1127-1139, 1975.

14. **Guarino, A. M., Anderson, J. B., Starkweather, D. K., Call J. B., and Oliverio V. T.,** Pharmacologic studies of camptothecin (NSC-100880): distribution, protein binding, and biliary excretion. *Cancer Chemother. Rep.* 57:125-140, 1973.

15. **Creaven, P. J. and Allen, L. M.,** Renal clearance of camptothecin (NSC-100880): effect of urine volume. *Cancer Chemother. Rep.* 57:175-184, 1973.

16. **Creaven, P. J., Allen, L. M., and Muggia, F. M.,** Plasma camptothecin (NSC-100880) levels during a 5-day course of treatment: relation to dose and toxicity. *Cancer Chemother. Rep.* 56:573-578, 1972.

17. **Horwitz, S. B., Chang C. -K., and Grollman, A. P.,** Studies on camptothecin: I. Effects on nucleic acid and protein synthesis. *Mol. Pharm.* 7:632-644, 1971.

18. **Horwitz, M. S. and Horwitz, S. B.,** Intracellular degradation of HeLa and adenovirus type 2 DNA induced by camptothecin. *Biochem. Biophys. Res. Comm.* 45:723-727, 1971.

19. **Horwitz, S. B., Chan, P., and Grollman, A. P.,** Studies on camptothecin. II. Antiviral activity. *Antimicrob. Agents & Chemotherap.* 2:395-401, 1972.

20. **Horwitz, S. B. and Horwitz, M. S.,** Effects of camptothecin on the breakage and repair of DNA during the cell cycle. *Cancer Res.* 33:2834-2836, 1973.

21. **Liebeskind, D., Horwitz, S. B., Horwitz, M. S., and Hsu, K. C.,** Immunoreactivity to antinucleoside antibodies in camptothecin treated HeLa cells. *Exper. Cell Res.* 86:174-178, 1974.

22. **Wall, M. E.,** Alkaloids with antitumor activity. In *Proc. Intl. Symp. Biochem. und Physiol. Alkaloide,* Berlin, June 28, 1969, Akademic Verlag, 77-87.

23. **Danishefsky, S., Quick, J., and Horwitz, S. B.,** Synthesis and biological activity in the camptothecin series. *Tetrahedron Letters.* 27:2525-2528, 1973.

24. **Bristol, J. A., Comins, D. L., Davenport, R. W., Kane, M. J., Lyle, R. E., Maloney, J. R., Portlock, D. E., and Horwitz, S. B.,** Analogs of camptothecin. *J. Med. Chem.* 18:535-537, 1975.

25. **Goldin, A., Venditti, J. M., and Mantel, N.,** Combination chemotherapy: basic considerations. In *Antineoplastic and immunosuppressive agents I.* Sartorelli, A. C. and Johns, D. G., Eds., Springer-Verlag, New York, 1974, 411-448.

26. **Moertel, C. G., Reitemeier, R. J., and Schutt, A. J.,** A phase II study of camptothecin (NSC-100880) in gastrointestinal cancer. *Proc. Am. Assoc. Cancer Res.* 12:18, 1971.

27. **Blaney, S. M., Balis, F. M., Cole, D. E., Craig, C., Reid, J. M., Ames, M. M., Krailo, M., Reaman, G., Hammond, D., and Poplack, D. G.,** Pediatric phase I trial and pharmacokinetic study of topotecan administered as a 24-hour continuous infusion. *Cancer Res.* (to be published, 1992).

28. **Shimada, Y., Yoshino, M., Wakui, A., Nakao, I., Futatsuki, K., Sakata, Y., Kambe, M., and Taguchi, T. A.,** Phase II study of CPT-11, a new camptothecin derivative, in patients with metastatic colorectal cancer. *Proc. Int. Symp. DNA Toposiomerases in Chemother.* Japanese Cancer Assoc., Nagoya, November 1991, 65.

29. **Sasaki, Y., Morita, M., Miya, T., Shinkai, T., Ekuchi, K., Tamura, T., Ohe, Y., and Saijo, N.,** Pharmacokinetic and pharmacodynamic analysis of CPT-11 and its active metabolite SN-38. *Amer. Soc. Clin. Oncol.* 11:111, 1992.

30. **Tanabe, R., Ikegami, Y., and Andoh, T.,** Inhibition of topoisomerase II by antitumor agents *bis*(2,6-dioxopiperazine) derivatives. *Cancer Res.* 51:4903-4908, 1991.

31. **Ishida, R., Miki, T., and Narita, T.,** Inhibition of intracellular topoisomerase II by antitumor *bis*(2,6-dioxopiperazines) derivatives: mode of cell growth inhibition distinct from that of cleavable complex-forming type inhibitors. *Cancer Res.* 51:4909-4916, 1991.

Preclinical Development of 20(*S*)-Camptothecin, 9-Aminocamptothecin, and Other Analogues

Milan Potmesil and Beppino C. Giovanella

CONTENTS

I. INTRODUCTION

Shortly after the establishment of structure-activity relationship among various semisynthetic and totally synthetic CAM derivatives,[1,2] and following the discovery of an overexpressed target DNA topoisomerase I (topo I) in advanced stages of human colon adenocarcinoma[3] and in other malignancies,[4] camptothecins were tested against human, inherently resistant cancers growing as xenografts in immunodeficient mice. Although the selected compounds have poor water solubility, their antitumor efficacy is better than that of water-soluble counterparts.

II. 20(*S*)-CAMPTOTHECIN

The initial discovery and chemical identification of 20(*S*)-camptothecin (CAM, NSC 94600), its testing against L1210 leukemia and Walker 256 carcinosarcoma, and the introduction of the water-soluble sodium salt (CAM-Na$^+$, NSC 100880) into clinical testing are discussed in Chapters 2 and 3 of this book. More recent tests in laboratory animals have shown a negligible antitumor activity of CAM-Na$^+$ even at levels substantially higher than the applied concentration of CAM.[5] The experiments and pharmacological studies, discussed in this chapter, have convincingly demonstrated the importance of the lactone form of camptothecins for effective cancer treatments.

CAM, isolated and purified from the plant, has poor water solubility. In biological studies, it becomes necessary to dissolve the substance in a strong organic solvent or formulate it as a suspension in Tween 80:saline or lipid media.[3,5,6] The type of formulation and the route of application has a considerable pharmacokinetic and pharmacodynamic impact. CAM suspension, injected subcutaneously (s.c.) or intramuscularly (i.m.) into immunodeficient nude mice, was tested using 14 human cancer xenograft lines.[5-7] Human cancer xenografts are a suitable model system, with elevated topo I levels comparable to the levels seen in surgical specimens of cancer tissues obtained from patients.[3,6] As mentioned earlier, water-soluble CAM-Na$^+$ was ineffective, while CAM treatment of tumor-bearing mice resulted in complete remissions in 11/14 lines such as lung (small and non-small cell), breast, ovary, pancreas, and stomach cancer and malignant melanoma. Gastrointestinal route was also used in the treatment of a lung adenocarcinoma and a melanoma xenograft line, and the treatments resulted in partial or complete remissions in most animals (Table 1). CAM was significantly more effective than any of clinically available anticancer drugs which were used as controls.[5] The drug suppressed the growth of central nervous system metastases of a malignant melanoma and lung adenocarcinoma xenografts.[6,7] The results of preclinical experiments were encouraging, and the compound was selected for clinical testing.

CAM in its lactone form can be isolated with cost effectiveness from natural sources and purified for trials in cancer patients. A single-institution clinical Phase I trial of CAM delivered orally was initiated in 1992, and the results are reported in Chapter 5.

III.   9-AMINO- AND 10,11-METHYLENEDIOXY CAMPTOTHECINS

Various semisynthetic or totally synthetic CAM analogues were prepared in the late 1970s and early 1980s either in a racemic mixture 20(RS) or as pure optically active 20(S) forms.[8–11] A number of compounds, with a good or poor water solubility, were tested for topo I-mediated DNA cleavage and cytotoxicity.[1,2] It was found that the analogues which induced accumulation of cleavable complexes in cells were effective in other topoisomerase I-directed screens and had good antitumor activity *in vivo*.[2] Among the drugs tested, 9-aminocamptothecin (9-AC, NSC 603071) and 10,11-methylenedioxycamptothecin (10,11-MDC) were selected for advanced testing and possibly clinical development

A twice-a-week schedule of 9-AC or 10,11-MDC injected s.c. or i.m. for 5–6 weeks had minimal toxicity and induced complete remissions of several human cancers including four lines of adenocarcinoma of the colon, infiltrating duct carcinoma of the breast, and malignant melanoma, all carried as xenografts in nude mice.[3,6,7,12] The lines, except breast cancer, were totally resistant to ten clinically available chemotherapeutics. 9-AC was effective not only in mice with small (0.2–0.25 cm^3 in size) but also with bulky tumors (average 2.5 or 8.0 cm^3). In some tumor lines, single-course treatment induced complete remissions which lasted over the life-span of experimental animals.[6] Drug treatment of experimental liver metastases was also studied. While the effect of a commonly used drug 5-fluorouracil was marginal at best, 9-AC prolonged the survival of treated mice significantly.[6,7,13] Given via gastrointestinal tract, 9-AC was fully active and induced, at somewhat higher doses, complete remissions of human cancer xenografts (Table 2).[14]

The results observed in experiments with 9-AC were comparable to those seen in CAM experimental treatments. However, 9-AC achieved the onset of a complete remission with lower total dose and within a shorter time period,[6,7,14] and a pattern of emerging resistance was seen in some mice carrying 3/14 cancer lines and treated with CAM, while there was no response failure among tumor-bearing mice treated with 9-AC.[6,7] Independent studies with human cancer xenografts conducted in several institutions[11,15] confirmed the original observation of 9-AC substantial efficacy.

Several 10,11-methylenedioxy analogues, namely 10,11-MDC, 9-amino-10,11-methylenedioxy-20(S)-camptothecin (9-A-10,11-MDC), and 9-chloro-10,11-methylenedioxy-20(S)-camptothecin(9-Cl-10,11-MDC), were synthesized and tested. Mechanistic studies show that the frequency of DNA-topo I cleavable complexes in a cell-free system and in treated cells induced by these analogues is, at equimolar concentrations, substantially elevated over the frequency induced by CAM or 9-AC.[16] The nonproliferating cells, such as B-lymphocytes obtained from patients with B-cell chronic lymphocytic leukemia (B-CLL), exposed to 10,11-MDC and triggered into proliferation, may be killed by a mechanism independent of DNA replication and resulting in the formation of irreparable DNA double-strand breaks.[17] In a clinically relevant study, a de-novo crossresistance to 10,11-methylenedioxy analogues was detected in B-lymphocytes

Table 1 **Intragastric treatment of BRO human melanoma xenografts with 20(*S*)-camptothecin**

mg/kg Dose	Application Schedule	Response T/A/P/C/*	Toxicity
—	—	6/2/0/0	—
1.5	weekdays	6/6/3/3	none
2.0	day 1,2 +, pause day 3	6/0/0/0	toxic deaths
2.0	day 1,2, +, pause day 3, 4	6/5/5/0	none
3.0	day 1 +, pause day 2	6/5/1/4	bw loss — 13%
3.0	day 1 +, pause day 2, 3	6/5/5/0	none

*Total number/Alive/Partial remission/Complete remission.

of approximately 13% of B-CLL patients.[17] Currently, these drugs are also tested in the xenograft model system.

Since 1989, 9-AC has been developed in collaboration between a research consortium and the Division of Cancer Treatments, National Cancer Institute. Limited water solubility, a property of some of the most active camptothecins, required pharmacological formulation suitable for clinical use. Bone marrow and gastrointestinal toxicities were dose-limiting in laboratory animals. Following pharmacokinetic studies and studies of drug formulation and toxicity, 9-AC entered a tri-institutional Phase I research as a 72-h continuous intravenous infusion (CIV) and a low-dose CIV escalated by time.[12,15]

IV. 9-NITRO-20(*S*)-CAMPTOTHECIN

Among various C9 substituents at the A ring of the CAM molecule, 9-nitro-20(*S*)-camptothecin (9-NC) is an intermediate of CAM synthetic conversion into 9-AC.[10] Since the yields of this semisynthetic product are higher than those of 9-AC, 9-NC has been considered for further development as an anticancer agent. As such, 9-NC was studied in the tissue culture, using normal and malignant human cell lines, and in human cancer xenografts. Although the *in vivo* studies are still ongoing, it appears that in resistant human cancer xenografts, such as colon adenocarcinoma or malignant melanoma, 9-NC is better than CAM but inferior to 9-AC.[6,7,12] In tissue culture experiments, 9-NC as well as CAM and 9-AC stopped the proliferating cells at the S-phase or G_2-phase of the cell cycle.[18–20] The S-phase arrest appeared as a prerequisite for programmed cell death.[21] The analogues were cytostatic for nontumorigenic cells but cytotoxic for tumorigenic cell lines.[18,19] This was shown in several tissue-culture lines which differed by their ability to induce tumors in immunodeficient mice.

Table 2 **Intragastric treatment of BRO human melanoma xenografts with 20(*S*)-camptothecin, 9-nitro-20(*S*), and 9-amino-20(*S*) camptothecins**

Drug	Dose mg/kg Single/Total	Application Schedule	Response T/A/P/C*	Toxicity
—	—	—	7/7/0/0	
CAM	1.0/15.0	weekdays	7/7/7/0	
9-NC	0.5/7.5	weekdays	7/7/7/0	
9-AC	0.5/7.5	weekdays	7/7/0/7	none

*Total number/Alive/Partial remission/Complete remission.

Normal human epidermal cells[22] and non-tumorigenic cells derived from human breast or ovarian cancer[18] exposed to 9-AC accumulate at the S/G_2 boundary. Upon drug removal, the cells re-enter the cell cycle. In contrast, S-phase tumorigenic cells of human malignant melanoma treated with 9-NC do not reach G_2 phase and die by apoptosis. Interestingly, low drug levels are more effective in the induction of irreversible programmed cell death than high drug concentrations.[22] This observation, if confirmed, may support the rationale for a low-dose continuous intravenous infusion (CIV) of camptothecins given to cancer patients (Chapter 9). The rationale for an alternative tapered-off CIV regimen, which is discussed in the following section, is supported by the conclusion that once the camptothecin-treated tumor cells enter the irreversible process of apoptosis, the continuous presence of the drug in culture media is not required.[22]

V. PHARMACOKINETIC AND PHARMACODYNAMIC STUDIES

Following an i.v. injection into a mouse, the radiolabeled CAM was almost ubiquitously distributed within 30 min, including the central nervous system, lungs, and the liver. A preferential accumulation of the drug, as seen in whole-body autoradiograms, was in the bile and the intestines.[23] In tissue-culture experiments, CAM, 9-AC, or 10,11-MDC entered the cells rapidly, and the level of cell-associated drugs remained elevated for 6 to 24 h over the drug level in tissue-culture media.[24,25] It is assumed that the lactone form remained reversibly bound to the cellular membrane system.[26] Comparative pharmacokinetic studies in the mouse have shown that the solubilized 9-AC, injected i.v., was rapidly eliminated from the body, while CAM and 10,11-MDC elimination was significantly slower.[27] Both latter drugs had substantially longer terminal half-life in plasma, and this is probably due to drug accumulation in peripheral tissues. The difference between 9-AC and CAM or 10,11-MDC, if confirmed in human, can be important for the selection of treatment schedules and routes of application.

Pharmacokinetics and pharmacodynamics of 9-AC was compared in the immunodeficient mice carrying human cancer xenografts.[12,28] It was shown that the solubilized 9-AC injected s.c. or i.m. was absorbed rapidly, and this was followed by a high plasma level of the active lactone form and by a rapid drug elimination with the terminal half-life of 1.58 h. Such treatment was toxic to the mouse, while the implanted tumors regressed only partially. At identical dose levels, the 9-AC suspension injected s.c. established a depot with gradual release of the drug into blood. The initial low peak of the 9-AC lactone in plasma was followed by gradual elimination with a terminal half-time in excess of 17 h. This treatment was without apparent toxicity and resulted in complete regressions of implanted tumors. The studies indicate that a low lactone plasma level, below the toxic threshold and sustained over extended time, is essential for optimal therapeutic effects. The tapered-off plasma level of 9-AC lactone form, with short intervals between the treatments, may significantly diminish the dose-limiting toxicities in normal tissues which have a low level of topo I expression, while preserving the cytotoxicity against the tumor tissue with overexpressed topo I.[12]

HPLC analytical methods have been devised for the detection of the lactone and the total drug level of CAM, 9-AC, and other analogues. The methods are applicable to plasma specimens obtained from patients treated with 9-AC or CAM.[24,25,27]

VI. CONCLUSIONS

The results obtained in the preclinical development of 9-AC and congeners are encouraging. Understandably, a more definite evaluation of CAM and analogues, in terms of their utility in cancer treatments, has to wait until more definite reports of clinical research become available.

Indications of a broad antitumor activity of 9-AC as well as CAM have been seen in the xenograft system. Although optimal schedules of administration may differ from one analogue to another, the reviewed preclinical study of the pharmacokinetics/ pharmacodynamics of 9-AC can provide leads. An effective treatment of resistant cancers in the xenograft system, such as advanced colon adenocarcinoma or non-small cell lung cancer, requires drug delivery over an extended period of time. To meet these ends in clinical research, several strategies should be explored: (1) A tapered-off CIV which provides for tapered-off plasma levels of the lactone form and results in preferential cytotoxicity against cancerous cells with overexpressed topo I. At the same time, this strategy may spare normal hematopoietic and mucosal progenitors with a low topo I level; (2) A low-dose CIV over a period of 21 days, currently used in Phase I/II trials of topotecan, may also provide for a differential cytotoxicity in a similar way as the tapered-off CIV does (see Chapter 9); (3) Since 9-AC and CAM are active when delivered orally, this route of application should be investigated; (4) Finally, preclinical research of dose-response relationship of camptothecins and combination additivity or synergism with alkylating agents will establish whether these drugs should be considered for high-dose chemotherapy with hematopoietic stem-cell support.

In the laboratory research discussed in Chapter 12, resistance to topo I-directed agents was developed in tissue culture by adaptation to a camptothecin and/or by mutagenesis. Several cell lines are available with structural changes of topo I gene accompanied by decreased topo I expression and function. Since drug resistance is the main reason for treatment failure in cancer patients, laboratory research of this event should be extended to clinical situations. This requires monitoring of tumor specimens, obtained before and during camptothecin-based chemotherapy, for relevant indicators of resistance such as topo I content, function, and structural changes of the topo I gene. The role of suppressor or regulatory genes on topo I gene expression and drug resistance should also be explored.

The unprecedented preclinical effectiveness of 9-AC, CAM, and related drugs against major therapy-resistant cancers warrants intensified laboratory and clinical research. Although unique features of topo I biology, biochemistry, and genetics have been explored, additional aspects of camptothecin-topo I-DNA interaction remain to be investigated. A high-resolution analysis of topo I quaternary structure by nuclear magnetic resonance or x-ray crystallography may provide not only an insight into the biochemistry of the enzyme inhibition by a camptothecin, but it can also be used for a rational design of effective analogues not cross-resistant with current topo I inhibitors.

ACKNOWLEDGMENTS

Supported in part by USPHS grants PO1 CA 50529, RO1 CA 54484, RO1 56129 and T32 HL 07151 from the National Cancer Institute, National Institutes of Health, and by a grant from the Stehlin Foundation for Cancer Research, the Friends of the Stehlin Foundation, and the Maria Slater Society for Research of Leukemia.

REFERENCES

1. **Jaxel, C., Kohn, K. W., Wani, M. C., Wall, M. E., and Pommier, Y.,** Structure-activity study of the actions of camptothecin derivatives on mammalian topoisomerase I. Evidence for a specific receptor site and for a relation to antitumor activity. *Cancer Res.,* 49: 1465–1469, 1989.
2. **Hsiang, Y.-H., Liu, L. F., Wall, M. E., Wani, M. C., Kirschenbaum, S., Silber, R., and Potmesil, M.,** DNA topoisomerase I-mediated DNA cleavage and cytotoxicity of camptothecin analogues. *Cancer Res.,* 49: 4385–4389, 1989.

3. **Giovanella, B. C., Stehlin, J. S., Wall, M. E., Wani, M. C., Nicholas, A. W., Liu, L. F., Silber, R., and Potmesil, M.,** DNA topoisomerase I-targeted chemotherapy of human colon cancer in xenografts. *Science,* 246: 1046, 1989.

4. **Potmesil, M., Hsiang, Y.-H., Liu, L. F., Bank, B., Grossberg, H., Kirschenbaum, S., Forlenzar, T. J., Penziner, A., Kanganis, D., Knowles, D., Traganos, F., and Silber, R.,** Resistance of human leukemic and normal lymphocytes to drug-induced DNA cleavage and low levels of DNA topoisomerase II. *Cancer Res.,* 48: 3537, 1988.

5. **Giovanella, B. C., Hinz, H. R., Kozielski, A. J., Stehlin, J. S., Jr., Silber, R., and Potmesil, M.,** Complete growth inhibition of human cancer xenografts in nude mice by treatment with 20-(*S*)-camptothecin. *Cancer Res.,* 51: 3052–3055, 1991.

6. **Potmesil, M., Giovanella, B. C., Liu, L. F., Wall, M., E., Silber, R., Stehlin, J. S., Jr., Hsiang, Y.-H., and Wani, M. C.,** Preclinical studies of DNA topoisomerase I-targeted 9-amino and 10,11-methylenedioxy camptothecins. In Potmesil, M. and Kohn, K. W., Eds., *DNA Topoisomerases in Cancer,* Oxford University Press, New York, 1991, 299.

7. **Potmesil, M., Giovanella, B. C., Wall, M. E., Liu, L. F., Silber, R., Stehlin, J. S., Wani, M. C., and Hochster, H.,** Preclinical and clinical development of DNA topoisomerase I inhibitors in the United States. In Andoh, T., Ikeda, H., and Oguro, M., Eds., *Molecular Biology of DNA Topoisomerases and its Application to Chemotherapy,* CRC Press, Nagoya, Japan, 1993, chap. 29, 301–311.

8. **Wall, M. E., Wani, M. C., Natschke, S. M., and Nicholas, A. W.,** Plant antitumor agents. 22. Isolation of 11-hydroxycamptothecin from *Camptotheca acuminata* Decne: total synthesis and biological activity. *J. Med. Chem.,* 29: 1553, 1986.

9. **Wani, M. C., Nicholas, A. W., Manikumar, G., and Wall, M. E.,** Plant antitumor agents. 25. Total synthesis and anti-leukemic activity of ring A-substituted camptothecin analogues. Structure-activity correlations. *J. Med. Chem.,* 30: 1774, 1987.

10. **Wani, M. C., Ronman, P. E., Moore, L., Truesdale, A., Leither, P., Lindley, J. T., and Wall, M. E.,** Plant antitumor agents. 18. Synthesis and biological activity of camptothecin analogues. *J. Med. Chem.,* 23: 554–560, 1980.

11. **Wall, M. E., Wani, M. C., Nicholas, A. W., Manikumar, G., Tele, C., and Besterman, J. M.,** Plant antitumor agents 30. Synthesis and structure activity of novel camptothecin analogues. *J. Med. Chem.,* 36: 2689–2701, 1993.

12. **Potmesil, M., Giovanella, B. C., and Wall, M. E.,** Unpublished results, 1994.

13. **Potmesil, M., Hinz, H. R., Marcee, A., Vardeman, D., Stehlin, J. S., Wall, M. E., Wani, M. C., Silber, R., and Giovanella, B. C.,** Growth inhibition of human cancer metastases in the xenograft model by camptothecin [NCS 94600, CAM], 9-amino-[NSC 603071, 9-AC], and 9-nitrocamptothecin. *Proc. Amer. Assoc. Cancer Res.,* 33: 432, 1992.

14. **Giovanella, B. C., Wall, M. E., Wani, M. C., Silber, R., Stehlin, J. S., Hochster, H., and Potmesil, M.,** Efficacy of camptothecin [NSC 94600, CAM], 9-aminocamptothecin [NSC 603071, 9-AC], and 10,11-methylenedioxycamptothecin [NSC 606174, 10–11-MDC] in human cancer xenograft model. *Proc. Amer. Assoc. Cancer Res.,* 33: 432, 1992.

15. 9-AC Investigators Meeting Minutes. Investigational Drug Branch, Cancer Therapy Evaluation Program, Division of Cancer Treatment/National Cancer Institute, June 9, 1992.

16. **Costin, D., Shen, T., Wall, M. E., Wani, M. C., Canellakis, Z. N., Potmesil, M., and Silber, R.,** Possible mechanism for greater cytotoxicity of 10,11-methylenedioxy-20(*S*)-camptothecin and its 9-amino analogue against chronic lymphocytic leukemia. *Proc. Amer. Assoc. Cancer Res.,* 34: 328, 1993.

17. **Costin, D., Potmesil, M., Newcomb, E. W., El Rouby, S., Thomas, A., Drygas, J., Morse, L., and Silber, R.,** *In vitro* sensitivity to camptothecins in B-cell chronic lymphocytic leukemia with and without p53 gene mutation. *Blood, J. Amer. Soc. Hemat.,* 82: 43a, 162, 1993.

18. **Pantazis, P., Early, J. A., Kozielski, A. J., Mendoza, J. T., Hinz, H. R., and Giovanella, B. C.,** Regression of human breast carcinoma tumors in immunodeficient mice treated with 9-nitrocamptothecin:Differential response of nontumorigenic and tumorigenic human breast cells *in vitro. Cancer Res.,* 53: 1577–1582, 1993.

19. **Pantazis, P., Kozielski, A. J., Mendoza, J. T., Early, J. A., Hinz, H. R., and Giovanella, B. C.,** Camptothecin derivatives induce regression of human ovarian carcinomas grown in nude mice and distinguish between nontumorigenic and tumorigenic cells *in vitro. Cancer Res.,* 53: 863–871, 1993.

20. **Pantazis, P., Mendoza, J. T., Kozielski, A. J., Natelson, E. A., and Giovanella, B. C.,** 9-Nitrocamptothecin delays growth of U-937 leukemia tumors in nude mice and is cytotoxic or cytostatic for human myelomonocytic leukemia *in vitro. Eur. J. Haematol.,* 50: 81–89, 1993.

21. **Tsao, Y. P., D'Arpa, P., and Liu, L. F.,** The involvement of active DNA synthesis in camptothecin-induced G_2 arrest: Altered regulation of $p34^{cdc2}$/cyclin B. *Cancer Res.,* 52: 1823–1829, 1992.

22. **Pantazis, P., Early, J. A., Mendoza, J. T., DeJesus, A. R., and Giovanella, B. C.,** Cytotoxic efficacy of 9-nitrocamptothecin in the treatment of human malignant melanoma cells *in vitro. Cancer Res.,* 54: 771–776, 1994.

23. **Smith, P. L., Liehr, J. G., Ahmed, A. E., Hinz, H. R., Mendoza, J., Kozielski, A., Stehlin, J. S., and Giovanella, B. C.,** Pharmacokinetics of tritium labeled camptothecin in nude mice. *Proc. Amer. Assoc. Cancer Res.,* 33: 432, 1992.

24. **Potmesil, M., Canellakis, Z. N., Wall, M. E., Wani, M. C., Nicholas, A. W., Mani, M., and Silber, R.,** Pharmacokinetic studies of 9-amino-20(*S*)-camptothecin [NSC 603071]: Cellular partitioning. *Proc. Amer. Assoc. Cancer Res.,* 33: 433, 1992.

25. **Costin, D., Silber, R., Canellakis, Z. N., Morse, L., and Potmesil, M.,** Uptake of 20(*S*)-camptothecin (CAMP) and analogues by human colon cancer cells or by chronic lymphocytic leukemia. In *The Fourth Conference on DNA Topoisomerase in Therapy,* New York, 1992, 53.

26. **Burke, T. G., Staubus, A. E., and Mishra, A. K.,** Liposomal stabilization of camptothecin's lactone ring. *J. Amer. Chem. Soc.,* 114: 8318–8319, 1992.

27. **Supko, J. G. and Malspeis, L.,** Pharmacokinetics of the 9-amino and 10,11-methylenedioxy derivatives of camptothecin in mice. *Cancer Res.,* 53: 3062–3069, 1993.

28. **Supko, J. G., Plowman, J., Dykes, D. J., and Zaharko, D. S.,** Relationship between the schedule dependence of 9-amino-20(*S*)-camptothecin (AC; NSC 603071) antitumor activity in mice and its plasma pharmacokinetics. *Proc. Amer. Assoc. Cancer Res.,* 33: 432, 1992.

Chapter 5

Phase I Clinical Trial and Pharmacokinetics Results with Oral Administration of 20(S)-Camptothecin

*John S. Stehlin, Ethan A. Natelson, Hellmuth R. Hinz,
Beppino C. Giovanella, Peter D. de Ipolyi, Kim M. Fehir,
Thomas P. Trezona, Dana M. Vardeman, Nicholas J. Harris,
Alice K. Marcee, Anthony J. Kozielski, and Amado Ruiz-Razura*

CONTENTS

I. INTRODUCTION

The natural product camptothecin (CPT) was first isolated from the Chinese tree *Camptotheca acuminata*. The chemical demonstrated substantial antitumor activity when tested in L1210 leukemia[1] and other murine tumors. Because of this, the drug was tested in clinical trials.[2-5] The chemical form employed for these trials was the sodium salt of CPT,[2] chosen for its water solubility, which allowed intravenous drug administration. Testing camptothecin in this salt form showed little promise because of a high degree of toxicity and only little antitumor activity.[13] It was not until CPT and some of its derivatives proved to be inhibitors of the DNA uncoiling enzyme topoisomerase I [7-10] that interest in the drug was revived.

In 1989, we determined in our laboratory that derivatives of CPT induced complete regression of human colon cancer xenografts.[11] We also showed that some of these derivatives had potent anticancer activity against a large variety of human cancer xenografts. The tumors against which CPT was successfully tested included human lung, prostate, breast, colon, stomach, and ovarian carcinomas, as well as melanomas, lymphomas, and sarcomas.[6,12-15] We determined that the intramuscular route (i.m.) of drug administration was the most effective, leading to complete tumor regressions after only a short period of time. We further found that oral administration (p.o.) was almost as good as i.m., but that the intravenous route (i.v.) was far inferior.[16] In fact, the antitumor activity of intravenous CPT was observed only after using prolonged continuous infusions. CPT exists in an equilibrium between the native lactone form and its carboxylate salt (see

Figure 1 below), whereby the lactone ring is opened up and converted into an ionic species. This ionic species is formed rapidly when exposed to a basic environment, including blood. It has to be reiterated that only CPT in its native form carries antitumor activity. We have repeatedly shown that the salt has no anticancer activity and is very toxic to animals. This apparently happened in the 1960s in some of the clinical trials.

Toxicity studies were performed in mice, rats, dogs, and pigs. After chronic and acute administration of CPT, by the three routes mentioned above, the main toxicity observed was an inflammatory ileitis which was completely reversible. The dogs seemed to be particularly sensitive, showing severe diarrhea followed by dehydration. Pigs were much more resistant. The use of steroids enabled us to control the symptoms and allowed the use of higher doses of CPT. Several autopsies were performed on the recovered animals. These showed only some enlarged mesenteric lymph nodes. The only time that bone marrow depression could be seen was when animals had previous prolonged and severe intestinal toxicities. These were the only observed toxicities in the animals studied.

II. RESULTS AND DISCUSSION

A. PATIENT SELECTION CRITERIA

Thirty-two male and twenty female patients were part of the study (52 total). The patient age ranged from 27–75 years. A total of 281 three-week courses of therapy were completed (Figure 2). All patients were evaluated for toxicity. The number and types of tumors present included colon cancer (13 patients), breast cancer (8), melanoma (7), lung cancer (5), pancreatic cancer (3), prostate cancer (5), multiple myeloma (2), sarcoma (2), cervical cancer (1), cholangiole cancer (1), rectal cancer (1), laryngeal cancer (1), kidney cancer (1), Hodgkin's disease (1), and non-Hodgkin's lymphoma (1).

All patients had histologically documented malignancies with measurable metastatic growths. Each patient had undergone extensive prior treatment and was refractory to currently available therapy. Admission criteria included an ambulatory performance status 60% on the Karnofsky scale, a serum creatinine level of 2.0 mg/dl, total bilirubin of 2.0 mg/dl, total leukocyte count of 3000/μl with total granulocytes 1500/μl, platelet count of 100,000/μl, and hemoglobin concentration of 9.0 gm/dl. All patients with active infections, brain metastases, and those with cardiac or vascular disease requiring anticoagulant therapy were excluded. All prior chemotherapy, hormonal therapy, immunotherapy, or radiotherapy must have been discontinued for a minimum of three weeks prior entry into the study (six weeks for nitrosoureas or mitomycin C).

B. DRUG ADMINISTRATION

Camptothecin (CPT) was packaged in a gelatin capsule and taken orally once a day for 21 days followed by 7 days rest. Each patient took the capsule in the morning on an empty stomach, approximately one half hour before breakfast. It was recommended that the capsule be taken with citrus juice, thus lowering gastric pH and providing an ideal environment for the stabilization of the lactone form of the drug. A minimum of three patients received CPT at each dose level, which escalated along a modified Fibonacci scale. The dose levels given were 0.3, 0.6, 1.0, 1.5, 2.1, 2.8, 3.7, 4.9, 6.5, 8.7, 11.6, and 15.4 mg/m^2/d. After each dose escalation, patients that developed significant toxicity were transferred to a lower level and maintained there. A dose level was maintained for the duration of three weeks. Patients who exhibited WHO Grade 4 hematologic or a Grade 3 non-hematologic toxicity were taken off the study. Lower toxicities were handled by reducing the treatment level and maintaining it.

Blood chemistry profiles were performed weekly initially and then continued at three-week intervals if no clinical signs of toxicity appeared. Treatment remained on an outpatient basis with weekly visits for physical examination, blood counts, and chemistry

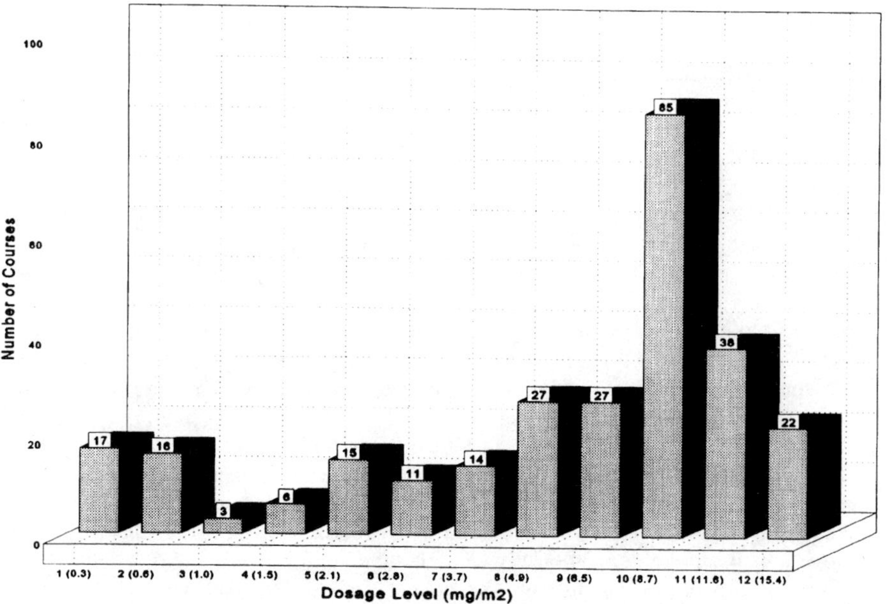

Figure 1 Shows relationship between camptothecin and its carboxylate salt. We have determined in our laboratory that the salt form of CPT is not only inactive but also very toxic to the animals and also to humans, as was shown during the clinical trials of the 1960s with CPT-sodium salt.

Figure 2 Number of courses given at each dosage level — 52 patients, 281 courses.

profiles. On occasion, chest roentgenogram and/or other scans were periodically reviewed to evaluate progress. A favorable response to CPT was assessed by assessing and measuring the shrinkage of tumor masses after a physical examination and by chemical or scanning techniques.

C. PLASMA LEVELS

The blood plasma concentration was analyzed for total CPT (plasma CPT plus CPT that was obtained by reconversion of the carboxylate salt into the lactone).[17] The reason for this methodology was that we determined that the actual amount of free CPT in the plasma was very sensitive to the speed of the workup, the reagents utilized, temperature applied to the sample, and solution volumes used. Plasma levels were determined by monitoring the fluorescence peak area. Excitation was set to 347 nm, and the emission was monitored at 418 nm. The measurements of plasma levels, determined in six patients, are exemplified in Figure 3. The figures follow a gradual accumulation over a period of 24 h until a steady state is reached.

D. PHARMACOKINETICS

The mean terminal half-life calculated for the drug compound was estimated to be 42 h $\pm$ 36 h. The mean maximum concentration of CPT in the blood was calculated to be 39 μg/ml $\pm$ 31 μg/ml. The mean AUC was determined to be 14 μg h/ml $\pm$ 23 μg h/ml.

Observable fluctuations in the value of the AUC are largely due to individual variability of patients and to the fact that the blood studies were carried out at different points during the treatment. It should be observed from Figure 1 that as soon as a dose of CPT is given, there is a sharp drop occurring in the CPT concentration. This drop is present from the beginning of treatment, and it becomes more pronounced the longer the patient is on the drug. This pattern, shown in Figure 1 could be observed with all patients. This observation suggests that CPT administration triggers a possible activation of enzymes, which remove CPT from the blood. It is interesting to observe that the drop is already measurable after the first dose of CPT and becomes more pronounced after the patients have been treated continuously for a longer period of time.

E. TOXICITY

All patients receiving more than 6.5 mg/kg/d had occasional loose stools. Persistent diarrhea was observed in only about 32% of the patients (Figure 4). Toxicities were generally manageable by symptomatic treatment with antidiarrheal medications. Only two patients required in-house admission as a direct result from diarrhea. The highest dose level that was best tolerated by most patients was 8.7 mg/m^2. Approximately 20% of patients experienced interstitial cystitis. The symptoms of cystitis resolved within a week of drug discontinuation but reappeared on occasion with continued administration. Cystoscopy in four patients disclosed erythema and rare, punctate mucosal ulcerations. Hematological toxicity was observed in only two patients who experienced granulocytopenia below 500/μl (WHO Grade 4) at a dose level of 2.8 mg/m^2. Both regained normal counts within 10–14 days. These two patients also experienced total alopecia coincident with the drop in white blood cell count. Both patients had been heavily pretreated with other anticancer drugs. No skin rashes, asthma, or other symptoms consistent with an allergic response were encountered. Twelve patients received CPT continuously from 6 to 12 months and five patients for more than one year. No long-term toxicities of any kind were observed.

F. ANTITUMOR ACTIVITY

Partial remissions were documented by physical examinations, laboratory workups, and radiographic scans. These occurred in two patients with breast cancer, two patients with melanoma, and one patient with prostate cancer. Three additional patients, one with lung cancer, one with melanoma, and one with breast cancer, exhibited stable disease for an extended period while on the drug. The most demonstrative response was observed in a patient with non-Hodgkin's lymphoma (diffuse, intermediate grade). At the onset of CPT therapy, he had generalized lymphadenopathy with axillary and inguinal lymph node masses, approximately 9 cm in diameter. He proved resistant to various protocols containing adriamycin, velban, cytoxan, corticosteroids, etoposide, bleomycin, vincristine, and

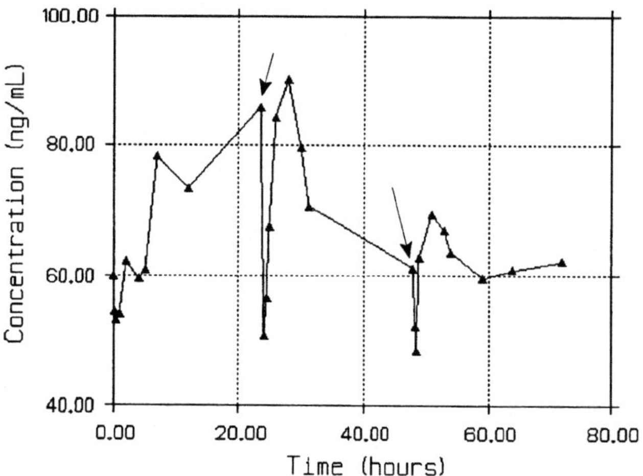

Figure 3 Graph shows plasma concentration of CPT in one patient who was pretreated with CPT for the duration of seven days. Arrows indicate the administration of the next dose. Note that the overall concentration of CPT is remaining relatively constant, indicating that a steady state has been achieved.

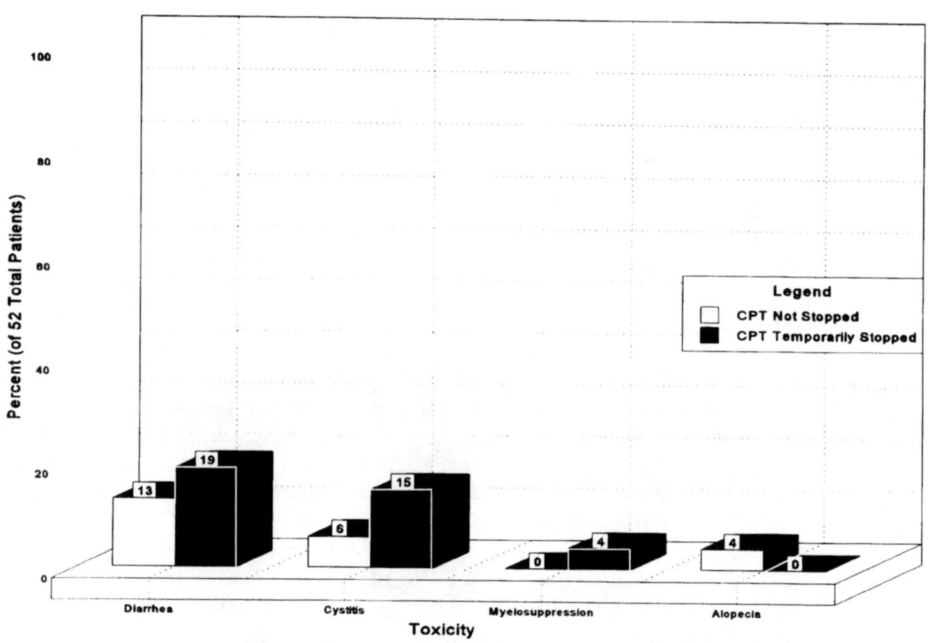

Figure 4 Toxicity studies.

cis-platinum. He remained in complete remission after one year of continuous treatment with CPT. He died four months after discontinuing CPT. Following an exploratory celiotomy for diverticulosis, no residual tumor was found.

III. CONCLUSION

Native 20(*S*)-camptothecin in the closed ring lactone form is a potent antitumor agent *in vitro* as well as *in vivo*. This chapter reports the clinical and pharmacokinetic results of administering 20(*S*)-camptothecin orally on a daily schedule. A total of 52 patients were treated, and a total number of 281 courses were given. Of these patients, six were chosen for pharmacokinetics studies. The dose range was from 0.3 to 15.4 mg/m^2. The maximum tolerated dose (MTD) that could be administered daily to almost all patients continually for several months was 8.7 mg/m^2. The plasma levels were determined by means of fluorescence. Pharmacokinetics calculations were fitted to the elimination curve to a biexponential model. The mean half-life was 42 hours with a standard deviation of ±36 hours. The area under the curve was 14 µg·h/ml ±23 µg h/ml. Clinically, diarrhea in about 32% of the patients was the primary toxicity followed by cystitis in about 20% of the patients. Both problems were completely reversible by discontinuation of the drug for a week. Only two heavily pretreated patients experienced granulocytopenia below 500/µl but recovered ten to fourteen days after discontinuing the drug. No long-term toxicities were observed. No patient died as a direct result from the drug. One complete remission and five partial remissions were reported. Furthermore, three patients showed stable disease for an extended period of time while being on the drug.

ACKNOWLEDGMENTS

The authors gratefully acknowledge the invaluable assistance of Mrs. Myrna Gibson for patient selection and the Friends of the Stehlin Foundation for Cancer Research for their financial support.

REFERENCES

1. **Wall, M. E., Wani, M. C., Cook, C. E., Palmer, K. H., McPhail, A. T., and Sim, G. A.,** Plant antitumor agents. I. The isolation and structure of camptothecin, a novel alkaloidal leukemia and antitumor inhibitor from *Camptothecin acuminata. J. Am. Chem. Soc.,* 88: 3888–3890, 1966.
2. **Gottlieb, J. A., Guarino, A. M., Call, J. B., Oliverio, V. T., and Block, J. B.,** Preliminary pharmacological and clinical evaluation of camptothecin sodium (NSC-100880). *Cancer Chemther. Rep.,* Part 1, 54: 461–470, 1970.
3. **Muggia, F. M., Creaven, P. J., Hansen, H. H., Cohen, M. N., and Selawry, O. S.,** Phase I clinical trials of weekly and daily treatment with camptothecin (NSC-100880). Correlation with preclinical studies. *Cancer Chemother. Rep.,* 56: 515–521, 1972.
4. **Gottlieb, J. A. and Luce, J. K.,** Treatment of malignant melanoma with camptothecin (NSC-100800). *Cancer Chemother. Rep.* 56: 103–105, 1972.
5. **Moertel, C. G., Schutt, A. J., Reitemeier, R. J. H., and Hahn, R. G.,** Phase II study of camptothecin (NSC 100880) in the treatment of advanced gastrointestinal cancer. *Cancer Chemother. Rep.,* 56: 95–101, 1972.

6. **Potmesil, M., Giovanella, B. C., Liu, L. F., Wall, M. E., Silber, R., Stehlin, J. S., Hsiang, Y.-H., and Wani, M. D.,** Preclinical studies of DNA topoisomerase I-targeted 9-amino and 10,11-methylenedioxy camptothecins. In Potmesil, M. and Kohn, K. W., Eds., *DNA Topoisomerases in Cancer,* Oxford University Press, New York, 1991, 299–311.

7. **Hsiang, Y.-H., Hertzberg, R., Hecht, S., and Liu, L. F.,** Camptothecin induced protein-linked DNA breaks via mammalian DNA topoisomerase I. *J. Biol. Chem.,* 260: 14873–14878, 1985.

8. **Hsiang, Y.-H. and Liu, L. F.,** Identification and mammalian DNA topoisomerase I as an intracellular target of the anticancer drug camptothecin. *Cancer Res.,* 48: 1722–1726, 1988.

9. **Jaxel, C., Kohn, K. W., Wani, M. C., Wall, M. E., and Pommier, Y.,** Structure-activity study of the actions of camptothecin derivatives on mammalian DNA topoisomerase-I: Evidence for a specific receptor site and a relation to antitumor activity. *Cancer Res.,* 49: 1465–1469, 1989.

10. **Hsiang, Y.-H., Liu, L. F., Wall, M. E., Wani, M. C., Nicholas, A. W., Manikumar, G., Kirschenbaum, S., Silber, R., and Potmesil, M.,** DNA topoisomerase I-mediated DNA cleavage and cytotoxicity of camptothecin analogues. *Cancer Res.,* 49: 4385–4389, 1989.

11. **Giovanella, B. C., Wall, M. E., Wani, M. C., Nicholas, A. W., Liu, L. F., Silber, R., and Potmesil, M.,** Highly effective topoisomerase I-targeted chemotherapy of human colon cancer in xenografts. *Science* (Washington, D.C.), 246: 1046–1048, 1989.

12. **Potmesil, M., Wall, M. E., Wani, M. C., Silber, R., Stehlin, J. S., and Giovanella, B. C.,** 9-Amino[NSC 629971, 9AC] and 10,11-methylenedioxy [NSC 606174, 10,11-MDC] camptothecins in the treatment of human cancer xenografts. *Proc. Am. Assoc. Cancer Res.,* 32: 337, 1991.

13. **Pantazis, P., Hinz, H. R., Mendoza, J. T., Kozielski, A. J., Williams, L. J., Jr., Stehlin, J. S., Jr., and Giovanella, B. C.,** Complete inhibition of growth followed by death of human malignant malanoma cell *in vitro* and regression of human melanoma xenografts in immunodeficient mice induced by camptothecins. *Cancer Res.,* 52: 3980–3987, 1992.

14. **Pantazis, P., Early, J. A., Kozielski, A. J., Mendoza, J. T., Hinz, H. R., and Giovanella, B. C.,** Regression of human breast carcinoma tumors in immunodeficient mice treated with 9-nitrocamptothecin: Differential response of nontumorigenic and tumorigenic human breast cells *in vitro. Cancer Res.,* 53: 1577–1582, 1993.

15. **Pantazis, P., Kozielski, A. J., Mendoza, J. T., Early, J. A., Hinz, H. R., and Giovanella, B. C.,** Camptothecin derivatives induce regression of human ovarian carcinomas grown in nude mice and distinguish between nontumorigenic and tumorigenic cells *in vitro. Int. J. Cancer,* 53: 863–871, 1993.

16. **Giovanella, B. C., Hinz, H. R., Kozielski, A. J., Stehlin, J. S., Silber, R., and Potmesil, M.,** Complete growth inhibition of human cancer xenografts in nude mice by treatment with 20-(S)-camptothecin. *Cancer Res.,* 51: 3052–3055, 1991.

17. **Stehlin, J. S., Natelson, E. A., Hinz, H. R., Giovanella, B. C., de Ipolyi, P. D., Fehir, K. M., Trezona, T. P., Vardeman, D. M., Harris, N. J., Marcee, A. K., Kozielski, A. J., and Ruiz-Razura, A.,** Phase I clinical trial and pharmacokinetic results with oral administration of 20(S)-camptothecin. Manuscript in preparation.

Clinical Studies of CPT-11 in Japan

Tetsuo Taguchi

CONTENTS

I. INTRODUCTION

Camptothecin is an alkaloid extracted originally from a plant, *Camptotheca acuminata*.[1] Camptothecin demonstrated antitumor activity *in vitro* and in experimental tumor systems, but its clinical application was discouraging because of inactivity and severe toxicities.[2] CPT-11, a semisynthetic derivative of camptothecin, was synthesized to impart aqueous solubility, greater antitumor activity, and less toxicity than camptothecin.[3] Camptothecin and its derivatives are attractive for cancer treatments since their new mechanism of action is the inhibition of topoisomerase I activity.[4]

Based on information from clinical phase I studies,[5,6] several phase II trials were started. New Drug Applications (NDA) have been filed in Japan for non-small cell lung cancers (NSCLC) and small cell lung cancers (SCLC), as well as uterine, cervical, and ovarian cancers. Some other studies including gastrointestinal, skin, and breast cancers, and hematological malignancies are also underway.

II. RESULTS OF PHASE I STUDIES

Two phase I studies were conducted to determine the maximum tolerated dose (MTD) and the dose limiting factor (DLF). CPT-11 was administered by drip infusion in both studies.[5] The results are summarized in Table 1.

In the single administration study in various tumors, DLF was leukopenia and MTD was presumed to be 250 mg/m^2 or more. Nadirs of leukopenia were obtained one week after the start of treatment, and it took 2 to 3 weeks for recovery. Thrombocytopenia and anemia were mild. Other main adverse reactions were nausea/vomiting, diarrhea, and alopecia, which were tolerable and reversible. The recommended dose of early phase II was 200 mg/m^2 every 3 or 4 weeks.

In another phase I study of weekly administration to patients with lung cancer,[6] DLFs were diarrhea and leukopenia with median time to nadir of 21 days, median recovery time

Table 1 **Results of phase I studies of CPT-11**

Item	Single Administration	Weekly Administration
Administration schedule	IV drip infusion for 30 min	IV drip infusion for 90 min
Target	Various tumors	Lung cancer
DLF	Leukopenia	Leukopenia, diarrhea
MTD	250 mg/m^2 or more	125 mg/m^2
Major adverse reactions	Leukopenia, anemia, thrombopenia, diarrhea, N/V, anorexia, alopecia	Leukopenia, anemia, thrombopenia, diarrhea, N/V, anorexia, alopecia
Recommended schedule for phase II study	200 mg/m^2/3–4 weeks	100 mg/m^2/week

of 7 days, and MTD of 125 mg/m^2. Other adverse reactions consisted of anemia, nausea/vomiting, anorexia, and alopecia. These were similar to those observed in phase I study of single administration. Therefore, weekly schedule for phase II study was recommended at a dose of 100 mg/m^2.

III. RESULTS OF PHASE II STUDIES

A. RESPONSE

1. Lung Cancer

A phase II study of patients with lung cancers was conducted with a regimen of weekly IV infusions at a dose of 100 mg/m^2.[8,9] The characteristics of eligible patients are shown in Table 2. Seventy-three previously untreated patients with NSCLC, 37 previously treated NSCLC, and 43 SCLC were enrolled, and out of these, 67, 26, and 35 patients, respectively, were evaluable for efficacy. Clinical responses were reviewed by extramural committees.

Table 2 **Patient characteristics**

	NSCLC		SCLC
	Untreated	Treated	
Eligible patients	73	36	41
(Evaluable for toxicity)	(72)	(35)	(39)
(Evaluable for efficacy)	(67)	(26)	(35)
Median age	67 years	58 years	62 years
(Range)	(34–75)	(38–70)	(40–74)
Sex: Male	53	22	33
Female	20	14	8
Stage I-II	3	2	1
IIIA	17	5	3
IIIB	13	8	8
IV	40	21	29
P.S. 0–1	54	23	28
2	19	13	13
Prior therapy			
No	73	0	8
Yes	0	36	33

Table 3 **Response of CPT-11 of patients with NSCLC (untreated)**

Histology	No. of Patients	CR	PR	MR	NC	PD	Response Rate (%) (CR + PR)
Adenocarcinoma	44	0	14	3	24	3	31.8
Squamous Cell	19	0	5	4	9	1	26.3
Large Cell	3	0	3	0	0	0	100
Adenosquamous	1	0	1	0	0	0	100
Total	67	0	23	7	33	4	34.3*

*95% confidence interval: 22.0–46.6%.

Table 4 **Response in SCLC**

Prior Therapy	No. of Patients	CR	PR	MR	NC	PD	Response Rate (%) (CR + PR)
No	8	0	4	0	2	2	50.0
Yes	27	2	7	0	13	5	33.3
Total	35	2	11	0	15	7	37.1*

*95% confidence interval: 19.3–54.9%.

Among 67 previously untreated NSCLC, 23 partial responses (PRs) and 7 minor responses (MRs) were observed with a response rate of 34.3%.The confidence interval of 95% was 22.0–46.6% (Table 3). CPT-11 was active against all major types of NSCLC. No responses were observed in previously treated NSCLC. There were 27 previously treated SCLC, and the response rate was 33.3% (9/27), including complete responses (CRs). In 8 previously untreated SCLC, the response rate was 50.0% (4/8). The overall response rate for SCLC was 37.1% (95% confidence intervals of 19.3–54.9%) (Table 4).

2. Gynecological Cancers

Clinical efficacy was studied in cervical and ovarian cancers with two @ regimens of weekly IV infusions at a dose of 100 mg/m^2 (Schedule A) and IV infusions every other week at a dose of 150 mg/m^2 (Schedule B).[10] The characteristics of eligible patients are shown in Table 5. Sixty-nine patients with cervical cancer and 75 ovarian cancer patients were enrolled, and the patients were allocated randomly to Schedule A or Schedule B. A total of fifty-five patients was evaluable for efficacy. For 55 evaluable cervical cancers, the response rate on Schedule A was 20.8% (5/24) with 2 CRs and 3 PRs and on Schedule B 25.8% (8/31) with 3 CRs and 5 PRs, showing no statistical difference in efficacy between the two schedules. The 95% confidence interval was 12.4–34.8% (Table 6). These responses were observed not only in squamous cell carcinoma but also in adenocarcinoma (Table 7). CPT-11 was active in distant metastatic lesions (20.9%, 9/43) including lung (28.6%, 6/21) and lymph nodes (25.0%, 2/8) as well as in primary tumors (25.0%, 3/12) (Table 8).

There were 36 previously treated ovarian cancer patients. Twenty-one had been treated with platinum(PT)-containing chemotherapies. The response rates in previously untreated, treated, and treated with PT were 31.6% (6/19), 19.4% (7/36), and 19.0% (4/21), respectively. Responses were also observed in patients with previous radiotherapy (26.8%, 11/14). The median dosage of CPT-11 for more than 50% tumor reduction was 425 mg/m^2 and the median duration of PR was 80 days.

Table 5   **Characteristics of patients with gynecological cancer**

	Cervical Cancer	Ovarian Cancer
Eligible patients	66	68
(Evaluable for toxicity)	(64)	(62)
(Evaluable for efficacy)	(55)	(55)
Median age	55 years	53 years
(range)	(22–74)	(27–75)
P.S.		
0–1	42	38
2–3	24	30
Primary	11	14
Recurrent	55	54
Prior therapy		
No	5	0
Yes	61	68
Radiotherapy	52	4
Chemotherapy	45	64
(with platinum)	(30)	(63)

Table 6   **Response of gynecological cancers by administration schedule**

Diagnosis	Method	No. of Patients	CR	PR	MR	NC	PD	Response Rate (%) (CR + PR)
Uterine cervical	A	24	2	3	5	4	10	20.8
cancer	B	31	3	5	2	11	10	25.8
	Overall	55	5	8	7	15	20	23.6*
Ovarian cancer	A	28	0	8	2	9	9	28.6
	B	27	0	5	2	9	11	18.5
	Overall	55	0	13	4	18	20	23.6*

Method A: Infusion intravenously at a dose of 100 mg/m^2 once a week. Method B: Infusion intravenously at a dose of 150 mg/m^2 once every 2 weeks. *95% confidence interval: uterine cervical cancer: 12.4–34.8%; ovarian cancer: 12.4–34.8%.

For 55 evaluable patients with ovarian cancer, the response rate on Schedule A was 28.6% (8/28) and on Schedule B 18.5% (5/27), showing no statistical difference. The 95% confidence interval was 12.4–34.8% (Table 6). These responses were observed in various histological types including serous cystadenocarcinoma, mucinous cystadenocarcinoma, endometric adenocarcinoma, and adenocarcinoma (Table 7). CPT-11 was active on both primary (20.0%, 1/5) and metastatic lesions such as intrapelvic (27.3%, 6/22) and intraperitoneal (25.0%, 4/16) and in distant metastatic lesions including the lung (25.0%, 1/4) and liver (25.0%, 3/12) (Table 9). It was noteworthy that 12 cases refractory to PT therapy showed clinical responses in 23.1% (12/52). The median dosage of CPT-11 to reach more than 50% tumor reduction was 400 mg/m,^{2} and the median duration of PR was 79 days.

3. Colorectal Cancer

Sixty-seven patients were enrolled. They were treated according to two regimens, Schedule A—100 mg/m^2 IV infusion once a week, Schedule B— 150 mg/m^2 IV infusion once

Table 7 **Response by histology**

Diagnosis	Method	No. of Patients	CR	PR	MR	NC	PD	Response Rate (%) (CR + PR)
Uterine	Squamous cell carcinoma	41	5	7	5	9	15	29.3
Cervical cancer	Adenocarcinoma	11	0	1	1	6	3	9.1
	Adenosquamous cell carcinoma	3	0	0	1	0	2	0
Ovarian cancer	Serous cystadeno-carcinoma	28	0	9	2	9	8	32.1
	Mucinous cystadeno-carcinoma	6	0	1	0	3	2	16.7
	Endometrioid adeno-carcinoma	8	0	1	1	3	3	12.5
	Clear cell adeno-carcinoma	8	0	1	0	1	6	12.5
	Undifferfentiated carcinoma	2	0	1	0	0	1	50.0
	Other	3	0	0	1	2	0	0

Table 8 **Response classified by lesion to uterine cervical cancer**

Evaluable Lesions	No. of Lesions	CR	PR	MR	NC	PD	Response Rate (%) (CR + PR)
Primary	12	0	3	0	6	3	25.0
Peripheral	19	3	4	2	4	6	36.8
Vagina	6	2	1	0	1	2	50.0
Others	13	1	3	2	3	4	30.8
Distant	43	5	4	7	11	16	20.0
Lung	21	5	1	4	6	5	28.6
Lymph node	8	0	2	2	2	2	25.0
Liver	6	0	0	1	1	4	0
Others	8	0	1	0	2	5	12.5

every two weeks.[11] Out of 67 patients, 53 were evaluable for efficacy including 60% of patients who had prior chemotherapy with 5-fluorouracil.

Overall response rate was 32.1% (17 PRs) (Table 10) and 42.3% (11/26) for the lung metastases and 20.0% (6/30) for liver metastases (Table 11).

4. Malignant Lymphoma

H. Tsuda, K. Ohta, T. Taguchi et al.[12] reported preliminary results in patients with malignant lymphoma. Fifty-nine patients with a lymphoma were treated with CPT-11 40 mg/m^2 IV infusion for 3 consecutive days repeated weekly, and 51 were evaluable for efficacy. Almost all patients had prior chemotherapies and relapsed after standard treatments.

The overall response rate (CR+PR) was 45.1%, and in non-Hodgkin lymphoma (NHL), 8 CRs and 15 PRs were observed (Table 12). All 8 patients with CRs had a previous relapse or refractory disease. The response rates for B-cell type NHL and T-cell

Table 9 **Response classified by lesion to ovarian cancer**

Evaluable Lesions	No. of Lesions	CR	PR	MR	NC	PD	Response Rate (%) (CR + PR)
Primary	5	0	1	2	1	1	20.0
Intrapelvic	22	0	6	2	9	5	27.3
Intraperitoneal	16	0	4	1	6	5	25.0
Distant	19	1	3	0	9	6	21.1
Lung	4	0	1	0	3	0	25.0
Liver	12	1	2	0	3	6	25.0
Others	3	0	0	0	3	0	0

Table 10 **Response to CPT-11 of patients with colorectal cancer**

Schedule	No. of Patients	CR	PR	MR	NC	PD	Response rate (%) (CR + PR)
A	24	0	7	0	9	8	29.2
B	29	0	10	2	8	9	34.5
Overall	53	0	17	2	17	17	32.1*

Method A: Infusion intravenously at a dose of 100 mg/m^2 once a week.

Method B: Infusion intravenously at a dose of 150 mg/m^2 once every 2 weeks.

*95% confidence interval: 19.5–44.7%.

Table 11 **Response classified by metastatic lesion to colorectal cancer**

Evaluable Lesions	No. of Lesions	CR	PR	MR	NC	PD	Response Rate (%) (CR + PR)
Lung	26	0	11	0	5	0	42.3
Lymph node	11	1	3	1	13	3	36.4
Liver	30	0	6	1	9	14	20.0

type NHL were 48.0% (12/25) and 57.1% (8/14), respectively. A 50% response rate (4/8) was observed in patients with adult T-cell leukemia/lymphoma.

B. MAIN ADVERSE REACTIONS

Main adverse reactions noted in late phase II clinical studies are shown in Table 13. These included myleosuppression and gastrointestinal symptoms (nausea, vomiting, diarrhea). Furthermore, the incidence of thrombocytopenia was low. All of these reactions were manageable and reversible.

The incidence of severely decreased WBC and hemoglobin was lower in patients with NSCLC and colorectal cancer than in patients with other cancer types. This is probably due to the absence of previous treatment and to the relatively early stage of the disease.

IV. CONCLUSION

CPT-11, a novel topoisomerase I inhibitor, is being studied clinically in Japan, Europe, and the United States. Japanese clinical investigations showed objective responses in non- small

Table 12 **Antitumor effect by disease**

Diagnosis	No. of Patients	CR	PR	MR	NC	PD	Response Rate (%) (CR + PR)
NHL	47	8	15	5	12	7	48.9
(ATL)	(8)	(1)	(3)	(0)	(2)	(2)	(50.0)
H D	4	0	0	0	1	3	0
Total	51	8	15	5	13	10	45.1*

*95% confidence interval: 34.4–55.8%.

Table 13 **Main adverse reactions in late phase II studies**

Diagnosis	WBC	Hb	Plt	Nausea/ Vomiting	Diarrhea	Alopecia
NSCLC	55.6	41.7	1.4	47.2	43.1	26.4
SCLC	82.1	51.3	7.7	35.9	35.9	25.6
Cervical cancer	89.1	50.0	10.9	51.6	39.1	38.1
Ovarian cancer	85.5	64.5	11.3	69.4	49.2	27.6
Colorectal cancer	54.8	35.5	4.8	50.8	31.7	44.4
Malignant lymphoma	87.0	47.8	26.1	50.0	60.7	10.9

Toxicity incidence (%) more than Grade 2 criteria (WHO).

cell and small cell lung, cervical, and ovarian cancers. Since major adverse reactions, including leukopenia and gastrointestinal toxicities, are reversible and clinically tolerable, CPT-11 is recommended for the treatment of patients with lung, gynecological, and colorectal cancers. Additional studies are showing clinical efficacy of CPT-11 in patients with malignant lymphoma.

REFERENCES

1. **Wall, M. E., Wani, M. C., Cook, C. E., Palmer, K. H., McPhail, A. T., and Sim, G. A.,** Plant antitumor agents 1. The isolation and structure of camptothecin, a novel alkaloidal leukemia and tumor inhibitor for *Camptotheca acuminata, J. Am. Chem. Soc.,* 88, 3888, 1966.
2. **Moertel, C. G., Schutt, A. J., Reitemeier, R., J., and Hahn, R. G.,** Phase II study of camptothecin (NSC-100880) in the treatment of advanced gastrointestinal cancer, *Cancer Chemother. Rep.,* 56, 95, 1972.
3. **Miyasaka, S., Sawada, S., Nokata, K., Sugino, E., and Mutai, M.,** New camptothecin derivatives, *Japan Kokai,* 19790, 1985.
4. **Hsaing, Y. H., Herzberg, R., Hecht, S., and Liu, L.,** Camptothecin induces protein-linked DNA-breaks via mammalian DNA-topoisomerase I., *J. Biol. Chem.,* 260, 14873, 1985.
5. **Taguchi, T., Wakui, A., Hasegawa, K., Niitani, H., Furue, H., Ohta, K., and Hattori, T.,** Phase I study of CPT-11, *Japan J. Cancer Chemother.,* 17, 115, 1990.
6. **Negoro, S., Fukuoka, M., Masuda, N., Takada, M., Kusunoki, Y., Matsui, K., Takifuji, N., Kudoh, S., Niitani, H., and Taguchi, T.,** Phase I clinical study of weekly intravenous infusion of CPT-11, a new derivative of camptothecin, in the treatment of advanced non-small cell lung cancer, *J. Natl. Cancer Inst.,* 83, 1164, 1991.

7. **Furuta, T. and Yokokura, T.,** Effect of administration schedules on the antitumor activity of CPT-11, a camptothecin derivative, *Japan J. Cancer Chemother.,* 17, 121, 1990.
8. **Negoro, S., et al.,** A phase II study of CPT-11, a camptothecin derivative, in patients with primary lung cancer, *Japan J. Cancer Chemother.,* 18, 1013, 1991.
9. **Fukuoka, M., et al.,** A phase II study of CPT-11, a new derivative of camptothecin, for previously untreated non-small cell lung cancer, *J. Clin. Oncology,* 10, 16, 1992.
10. **Takeuchi, S., et al.,** A late phase II study of CPT-11 on uterine cervical cancer and ovarian cancer, *Japan J. Cancer Chemother.,* 18, 1681, 1991.
11. **Shimada, Y.,** A phase II study of CPT-11, a new camptothecin derivative, in *Proc. Vth World Conference on Clinical Pharmacology and Therapeutics Highlights of a Satellite Symposium,* Taguchi, T. and Wang, J. C., Eds., PMSI Japan, 1992, chap. 8.
12. **Tsuda, H., Takatsuki, K., Ohno, R., Masaoka, T., Okada, K., Shirakawa, S., Ohashi, Y., Ohta, K., and Taguchi, T.,** A late phase II trial of potent topoisomerase I inhibitor, CPT-11, in malignant lymphoma, in *Proc. Am. Soc. Clin. Oncology,* 11, 1992, 316.

Chapter 7

Clinical Trials and Pharmacokinetic Studies of CPT-11 in the United States

*Mace L. Rothenberg, Eric K. Rowinsky, John G. Kuhn,
Howard A. Burris, III, Ross C. Donehower, and Daniel D. Von Hoff*

CONTENTS

I. INTRODUCTION

Camptothecin and its derivatives comprise a unique family of natural product compounds that has generated a great deal of excitement in the medical oncology community. Camptothecins stabilize the topoisomerase I-DNA cleavable complex and thereby interfere with DNA replication and transcription. No other antitumor compounds currently in use work in this fashion. CPT-11 is a water-soluble analog of camptothecin that was first synthesized in Japan in the early 1980s.[1-2] *In vitro*, CPT-11 was found to possess more potent antitumor activity than camptothecin, and Phase I clinical trials conducted in Japan in the mid-1980s confirmed that CPT-11 could be administered without the severe and unpredictable side effects that plagued the first clinical trials of camptothecin sodium. Recent reports from Phase II trials conducted in Japan have documented significant clinical activity of CPT-11 against a broad array of solid tumors, including small cell and non-small cell lung cancer, colorectal cancer, squamous cell carcinoma of the cervix, and ovarian cancer.[3-8] The reader is referred to Chapter 6 in this book for further details.

CPT-11 entered Phase I clinical trial in Europe and the United States in mid-1991. This report summarizes the results of U.S. Phase I trials.

II. TRIAL DESIGNS

Two Phase I trials have now been completed in the United States. Investigators at Johns Hopkins have explored a dosing schedule of one 90-min intravenous infusion administered every three weeks, while researchers at the University of Texas Health Science Center at San Antonio have performed a Phase I trial of CPT-11 given over 90 minutes IV weekly for four consecutive weeks followed by a two-week rest period. Both trials used standard Phase I patient eligibility criteria.

III. PATIENT CHARACTERISTICS

In total, 64 patients were entered and more than 200 courses of therapy were administered in these two Phase I trials of CPT-11. Doses explored in the q 3-week schedule ranged from 100–345 mg/m^2, while the weekly dosing schedule examined dose levels of 50–180 mg/m^2/wk. Patient characteristics were quite similar in both studies, with the majority of patients having received prior chemotherapy (29/32 in the San Antonio trial and 29/32 in the Hopkins trial). Patients received a median of two chemotherapy regimens prior to entering the CPT-11 Phase I trials. All patients in the Hopkins trial were ECOG performance status 0–1, while the San Antonio trial enrolled 28 of 32 such patients as well as four patients with a performance status of 2. Colorectal carcinoma accounted for 22 of the 32 patients in the San Antonio study and 12 of the 32 patients in the Johns Hopkins study. Other commonly represented tumors in the Phase I trials included non-small cell lung (7 patients) and cervix cancers (5 patients) at Hopkins and cervix (2 patients) and breast cancers (2 patients) at San Antonio.

IV. RESULTS

At Johns Hopkins, dose-limiting toxicity was encountered at the 290 and 345 mg/m^2 dose levels. It was manifested as Grade 4 neutropenia in one patient, nausea and vomiting persisting despite aggressive antiemetics in one patient, and Grade 4 diarrhea in one patient. There were no differences in the frequency or severity of these dose-limiting toxicities when comparing lightly pretreated (i.e., those with 0–2 prior chemotherapy regimens and no prior abdominal or pelvic radiation) to heavily pretreated (i.e., 3 or more prior chemotherapy regimens and/or prior abdominal or pelvic radiation) patients. For this reason, the maximum tolerated dose of CPT-11 on this schedule was determined to be 240 mg/m^2.[13]

At San Antonio, diarrhea was identified as the dose-limiting toxicity, occurring in three of the six individuals treated at the 180 mg/m^2 dose level. This Grade 4 diarrhea was accompanied by abdominal cramping and dehydration and required hospitalization for fluid and electrolyte support. While less severe cases of diarrhea were encountered sporadically at lower dose levels and controlled by aggressive use of loperimide and diphenhydramine, the diarrhea that occurred at the 180 mg/m^2 dose level was unaffected by loperamide, diphenhydramine, paregoric, Lomotil, or octreotide. Typically, the diarrhea remained severe for five to seven days before resolving. Prior chemotherapy or radiation did not seem to influence the frequency or severity of this toxicity; it was as common in lightly pretreated patients as it was in heavily pretreated patients. Due to this Grade 4 diarrhea, the maximum tolerated dose of CPT-11 on this weekly schedule was defined as 150 mg/m^2. Myelosuppression was not a major toxicity of CPT-11 in this trial; only 2.5% of all treatment cycles resulted in Grade 4 granulocytopenia (i.e., granulocytes < 500/μl). There was a trend toward more severe granulocytopenia in patients who had received prior abdominal or pelvic irradiation, but this was not statistically significant.[12]

Objective responses have been seen in both trials. Two partial responses have been described by the Johns Hopkins group. One patient with metastatic colorectal carcinoma who was treated at the 240 mg/m^2 dose level experienced resolution of right upper quadrant pain, a 95% decrease in the size of measurable hepatic lesions, and normalization of CEA. This response has persisted for 11+ months. The other partial response was observed in a patient with squamous cell carcinoma of the cervix who was treated at the 290 mg/m^2 level. Lymph node metastases decreased by more than 80%, and this response has lasted for 5+ months. Each of these patients had received previous treatment: multiple 5-FU-based chemotherapy regimens for the patient with colon cancer and pelvic irradiation and combination chemotherapy for the patient with cervical cancer.

In San Antonio, there have been two partial responses, both occurring in patients with metastatic colorectal carcinoma that had recurred following treatment with multiple 5-FU-based regimens. One patient treated at the 80 mg/m^2 dose level had a greater than 80% shrinkage in tumor dimensions that lasted for eight months. Another patient treated at the 125 mg/m^2 dose level had tumor shrinkage of greater than 90% that persisted for ten months. Both patients remained fully active throughout the course of CPT-11 treatment.

V. PHARMACOKINETIC STUDIES

In San Antonio, serial blood and urine samples were collected from at least two patients treated at each dose level. Samples were obtained during and after the first dose of CPT-11. A reverse-phase high performance liquid chromatography (HPLC) assay, developed by Kaneda and colleagues, was used to measure CPT-11 and SN-38.[9] CPT-11 and its active metabolite, SN-38, occur in two forms: the lactone (active) and carboxylate (inactive) forms. A pH-dependent equilibrium exists between the lactone and carboxylate species, with acidic pH driving the reaction toward the lactone and basic pH moving the reaction toward the carboxylate. Our assay measured lactone and total levels of CPT-11 and SN-38. A typical example of the plasma elimination curves for these compounds is depicted in Figure 1. Peak plasma concentration of CPT-11 occurred at the end of infusion, while peak concentrations for SN-38 were more variable, occurring 30–90 minutes after the end of infusion. Both CPT-11 and SN-38 undergo biexponential elimination. Over all dose levels tested, the mean terminal half-life of CPT-11 (total) was 7.9 ± 2.8 hours, while for the CPT-11 (lactone), the mean terminal $t_{1/2}$ was 6.3 ± 2.2 hours. For the SN-38, the mean terminal half-life was 13.0 ± 5.8 hours for the total and 11.5 ± 3.8 for the lactone. There was a strong linear relationship between dose and CPT-11 peak plasma concentration ($C_p$max) as well as CPT-11 dose and area under the concentration curve (AUC) (Figures 2a and 2b). There was no relationship noted between CPT-11 dose and SN-38 $C_p$max or AUC.

Renal excretion does not appear to be the primary route of elimination for either CPT-11 or SN-38. As shown in Table 1, only 13.9 ± 6.5% of CPT-11 and 0.26 ± 0.19% of SN-38 were recovered from the urine over the 48 hours during and immediately following CPT-11 administration.

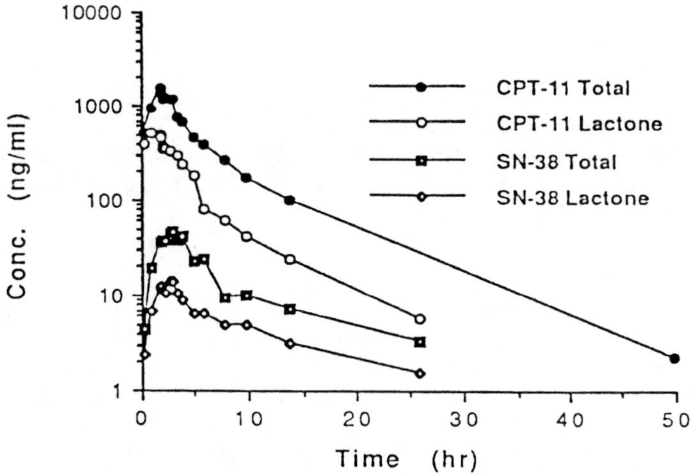

Figure 1 Plasma elimination curve for CPT-11 and SN-38 in a representative patient treated at the 150 mg/m^2 dose level (San Antonio trial).

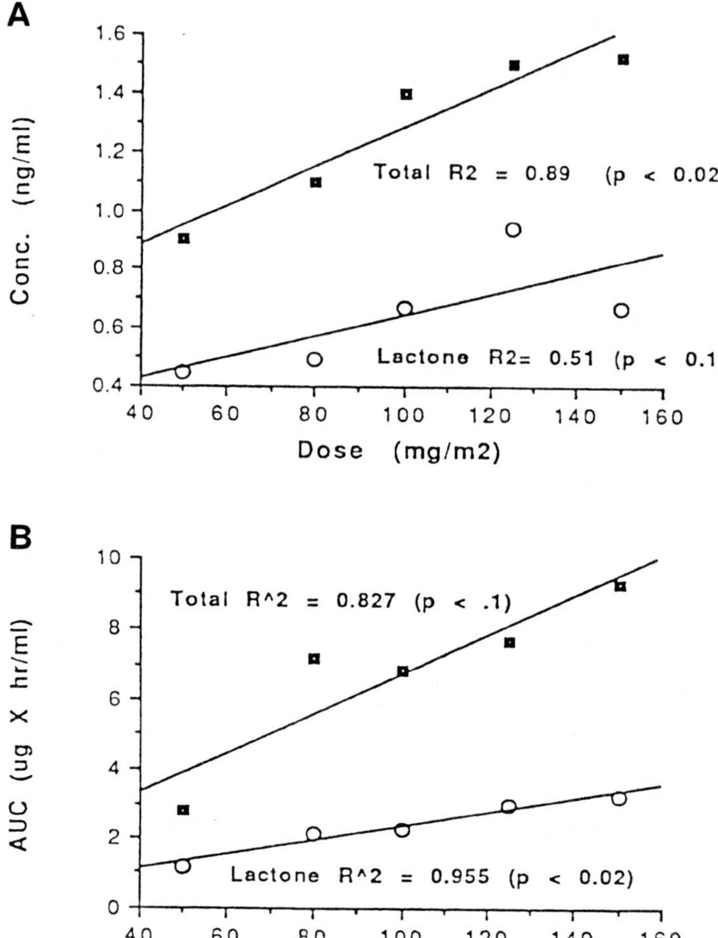

Figure 2 (a) Peak plasma concentration of CPT-11 as a function of CPT-11 dose. **(b)** Area under the concentration curve for CPT-11 as a function of CPT-11 dose. Total CPT-11 represented by solid squares (■), and lactone ring form represented by open circles (○) (San Antonio trial).

Prior to initiation of treatment with CPT-11, one patient with colon cancer developed biliary obstruction as a result of a large metastasis in the porta hepatis. Percutaneous biliary drainage was required. The hyperbilirubinemia resolved, and this patient was subsequently treated at the 100 mg/m^2/wk dose level. Plasma and bile samples obtained during and immediately following CPT-11 administration demonstrated bile-to-plasma ratios as high as 60:1 for CPT-11 and 9:1 for SN-38 (Figure 3). The high concentrations of CPT-11 and SN-38 found in the bile suggest that biliary excretion is an important, if not primary, route of clearance for these compounds.

Table 1 **CPT-11/SN-38 urinary excretion**

PT. #	Dose (mg/m²)	% Urinary Excretion CPT-11	Over 48 Hrs. SN-38
1	50	2.5	0.13
2	50	16.9	0.29
3	80	8.9	0.09
4	80	10.1	0.15
5	100	7.3	0.08
6	100	18.6	0.60
7	100	18.5	0.11
8	125	21.5	0.37
9	125	21.1	0.52
10	150	14.3*	0.25*
Mean (n = 9)		13.9	0.26
± SD		(6.5)	(0.19)

*Incomplete collection.

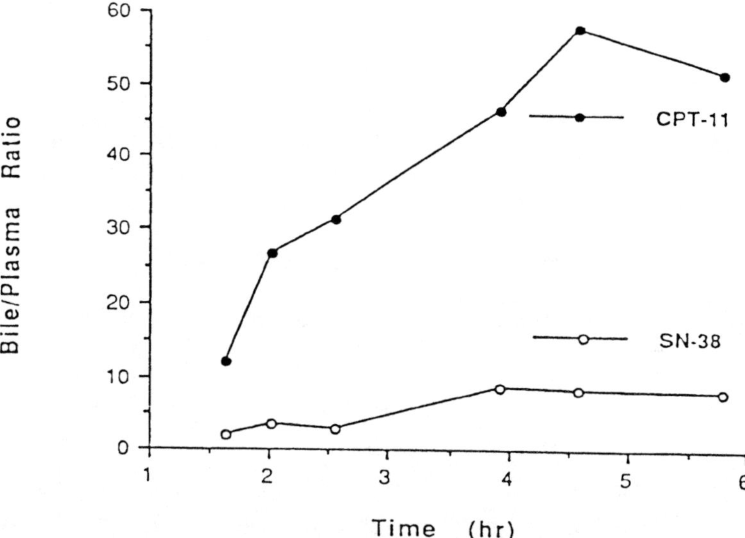

Figure 3 Bile-to-plasma concentration ratio for CPT-11 (●) and SN-38 (○) (San Antonio trial).

VI. CONCLUSIONS

CPT-11 is a water-soluble camptothecin derivative that has demonstrated significant antitumor activity *in vitro* and *in vivo*. CPT-11 is converted by endogenous carboxylesterases in the liver, gastrointestinal tract, and blood to SN-38. This metabolite is 200–1000 times more potent than CPT-11 in the inhibition of topoisomerase I activity.[10] *In vitro*, intracellular SN-38 appears to account for most, if not all, of the DNA strand breaks that are observed following exposure to CPT-11. In fact, some consider CPT-11 to be a prodrug for SN-38.

Phase I evaluation of CPT-11 has now been completed in the United States. In the Phase I trial conducted at Johns Hopkins, the maximum tolerated dose for CPT-11 given on a q three-week schedule was 240 mg/m^2. The San Antonio Phase I trial identified 150 mg/m^2 as the MTD when CPT-11 was given on a weekly $\times$ 4 basis, followed by a two-week rest. Dose-limiting toxicity for the weekly schedule was diarrhea, while DLT on the q three-week schedule was diarrhea, as well as nausea, vomiting, and neutropenia. The etiology for this diarrhea is unclear, but early recognition and intervention with supportive measures appear to be crucial in its management. There were no specific patient characteristics that were useful in identifying those patients at highest risk of developing Grade 4 diarrhea. Neither extent of prior therapy, history of pelvic irradiation, tumor type, tumor location, age, or sex of the patient proved useful in predicting which patients would experience this GI toxicity. Future efforts will need to determine whether any pharmacokinetic parameters correlate reliably with diarrhea.

Pharmacokinetic analysis performed in conjunction with the San Antonio trial revealed that CPT-11 and SN-38 have relatively long terminal half-lives. This can be considered a favorable characteristic for a drug whose mechanism of action is primarily directed against cells in the DNA-synthesis phase of the cell cycle. Neither CPT-11 nor SN-38 appears to be primarily cleared by the kidney, but significant bile-to-plasma concentration gradients were found in one patient. This is in agreement with preclinical data from the mouse that suggest that biliary clearance is the major route of excretion for CPT-11 and SN-38.[11] One may speculate that concentration of these compounds in the liver, bile, and gastrointestinal tract may contribute to antitumor activity against malignancies that affect these organs.

In the San Antonio trial, a significant correlation was found between CPT-11 dose, peak plasma concentration, and area under the concentration curve. No such relationship was found to exist between SN-38 pharmacokinetics and CPT-11 dose. One possible explanation for this variability in SN-38 pharmacokinetics might be carboxylesterase polymorphism, but direct studies are needed to confirm this hypothesis.

Overall, four objective responses were observed in these two trials: three in patients with recurrent colorectal cancer and one in a patient with recurrent squamous cell carcinoma of the cervix. This is consistent with the antitumor activity reported in Phase I and II trials from Japan. In followup, Phase II trials have now begun in the United States to evaluate the antitumor activity of single agent CPT-11 in patients with recurrent colorectal and cervical cancers. Future clinical trials are likely to proceed along two parallel tracks: additional single-agent Phase II trials to examine the activity of CPT-11 against other tumor types (e.g., small cell and non-small cell lung cancer, ovarian cancer) and CPT-11-based drug combination studies to identify additive or synergistic activity of CPT-11 when used in conjunction with other drugs (e.g., 5-FU and leucovorin in the treatment of colorectal cancer or cisplatin in the treatment of lung cancer). It is only through this type of broad approach that the full benefit of CPT-11 will be realized.

ACKNOWLEDGMENTS

The authors would like to acknowledge Kiyoshi Terada, Ph.D., of Yakult Honsha Co., Ltd., and Michael K. Rock, Pharm.D., of G.H. Besselaar Associates for their support of this trial.

REFERENCES

1. **Yokokura, T., Sawada, S., Nokata, K., et al.,** Antileukemic activity of new camptothecin derivatives. In *Proc. Japanese Cancer Assoc.,* 40th Ann. Meet., Sapporo, Japan, 228 (1981).
2. **Yokokura, Furata, Sawada, S., et al.,** Antitumor activity of newly synthesized, lactone ring-closed and water-soluble camptothecin derivative in mice. In *Proc. Japanese Cancer Assoc.,* 43rd Ann. Meet., Fukuoka, Japan, 261 (1984).
3. **Negoro, S., Fukuoka, M., Masuda, N., et al.,** Phase I study of weekly intravenous infusions of CPT-11, a new derivative of camptothecin, in the treatment of advanced non-small cell lung cancer. *J. Natl. Cancer Inst.,* 83:1164-1168, 1991.
4. **Masuda, N., Fukuoka, M., Takada, M., et al.,** CPT-11 in combination with cisplatin for advanced non-small cell lung cancer. *J. Clin. Oncol.,* 10:1775-1780, 1992.
5. **Masuda, N., Fukuoka, M., Kusunoki, Y., et al.,** CPT-11: a new derivative of camptothecin for the treatment of refractory or relapsed small cell lung cancer. *J. Clin. Oncol.,* 10:1225-1229, 1992.
6. **Takeuchi, S., Noda, K., Yakushiji,** and CPT-11 Study Group in Gynecologic Malignancy, Late phase II study of CPT-11, topoisomerase I inhibitor, in advanced cervical carcinoma. *Proc. Am. Soc. Clin. Oncol.,* 11:224, 1992.
7. **Shimada, Y., Yoshino, M., Wakui, A., et al.,** Phase II study of CPT-11, new camptothecin derivative, in the patients with metastatic colorectal cancer. *Proc. Am. Soc. Clin. Oncol.,* 10:135, 1991.
8. **Takeuchi, S., Takamizawa, H., Takeda, Y., et al.,** Clinical study of CPT-11, camptothecin derivative, on gynecologic malignancy. *Proc. Am. Soc. Clin. Oncol.,* 10:189, 1991.
9. **Kaneda, N. and Yokokura, T.,** Nonlinear pharmacokinetics of CPT-11 in rats. *Cancer Res.,* 50:1721-1725, 1990.
10. **Kawato, Y., Aonuma, M., Hirota, Y., et al.,** Intracellular roles of SN-38, a metabolite of the camptothecin derivative CPT-11, in the antitumor effect of CPAT-11. *Cancer Res.,* 51:4187-4191, 1991.
11. Investigators Brochure, *CPT-11.* G.H. Besselaar Associates, 1991.
12. **Rothenberg, M. L., Kuhn, J. G., Burris, H. A., III, et al.,** Phase I and pharmacokinetic trial of weekly CPT-11. *J. Clin. Oncol.,* 11:2194-2204, 1993.
13. **Rowinsky, E., Grochow, L., Ettinger, D., et al.,** Phase I and pharmacologic study of CPT-11, a semisynthetic topoisomerase I-targeting agent, on a single-dose schedule. *Proc. Am. Soc. Clin. Oncol.,* 11:115, 1992 (abstract #281).

Chapter 8

Clinical Trials and Pharmacology Studies of CPT-11 and its Active Metabolite SN-38 in France: Preliminary Pharmacokinetic-Pharmacodynamic Relationships

*Guy G. Chabot, Marcel de Forni, Daniel Abigerges,
Jean-Pierre Armand, Michel Clavel, Roland Bugat, Stéphane Culine,
Jean-Marc Extra, Michel Marty, Marie-Christine Bissery,
Anne Mathieu-Boué, Patrice Hérait, and Alain Gouyette*

CONTENTS

I. INTRODUCTION

CPT-11 (irinotecan) is a semisynthetic derivative of camptothecin[1-9] that was selected for clinical testing based on its improved water solubility and its good *in vitro* and *in vivo* activity in various experimental systems, including pleiotropic drug-resistant tumors (see Chapter 1 for structure).[10-14] As with the parent compound camptothecin,[15,16] the mechanism of action of CPT-11 is presumed to be mediated through topoisomerase I inhibition.[17]

Prior Japanese Phase I and II studies have shown encouraging response rates in non-small cell lung cancer, refractory leukemia and lymphoma, small cell lung cancer, colon cancer, and gynecological cancer.[18-22]

In 1990, Phase I studies have been initiated in France using three different schedules in an attempt to determine the optimal administration scheme for CPT-11: daily for three consecutive days every three weeks,[23] weekly for three weeks,[24] and once every three weeks.[25]

To understand CPT-11 clinical pharmacology better and examine pharmacokinetic-pharmacodynamic relationships that could be useful in the future clinical management of this drug, we determined the pharmacokinetics of both CPT-11 and its active metabolite SN-38 during the three French Phase I clinical trials. We report here the preliminary findings of these pharmacological studies.

II. PATIENTS AND METHODS

A. PATIENTS

As of February 1992, 152 patients refractory to conventional therapy were entered in three Phase I studies.[23-25] All patients had to meet the following standard Phase I eligibility criteria:

1. Histologically confirmed malignant solid tumor, refractory to standard therapy, or for which no established therapy is available;
2. No chemotherapy or radiotherapy four weeks before entry (six weeks for nitrosoureas and mitomycin C);
3. Age between 18 and 75 years;
4. Performance status of 0–2, according to WHO scale;
5. Life expectancy of at least three months;
6. Adequate hematological parameters (WBC $\geq$ 4000/μl, platelet count $\geq$ 100,000/μl, and hemoglobin $\geq$ 10 g/dl), hepatic function (bilirubin and transaminase level $\leq$ 2 $\times$ upper limit of normal values), and renal function (creatinine $\leq$ 120 μmol/l);
7. No evidence of cardiac dysfunction;
8. No previous anaphylactic reactions;
9. A signed consent form obtained for all patients.

Prior to the first CPT-11 course, each patient had a medical history, physical examination, complete blood cell count, serum chemistry for electrolytes, renal and hepatic functions, urinalysis, and chest X-ray. The complete blood cell counts were repeated at least twice weekly, and other biological tests were performed once a week.

B. ASSESSMENT OF TOXICITY AND EFFICACY

The toxic effects and tumor responses were classified according to the WHO criteria.[26]

C. DRUG ADMINISTRATION

CPT-11 was administered according to three different schedules: daily for three consecutive days every three weeks, weekly for three weeks, and once every three weeks. CPT-11 was provided by Yakult Honsha Co., Ltd., (Tokyo, Japan) as a solution ready for use, in 2- or 5-ml vials containing 40 and 100 mg of the drug, respectively. The required dose was further diluted in 250 ml of 0.9% sodium chloride in water and administered as a 30-min IV infusion into a peripheral vein.

D. PHARMACOKINETICS

Heparinized blood samples (2 ml) were collected immediately before the infusion time (time 0) and at the following times thereafter: 10, 20, and 30 min during the 30-min IV infusion; after the infusion at 5, 10, 15, 30, 45, and 60 min; then at 2, 4, 8, 12, and 24 h post-infusion. In many patients, sampling was prolonged up to 48 h. Blood was immediately centrifuged at 2000 $\times$ g for 15 min, and the plasma was transferred to a 1.5 ml polypropylene tube, frozen and kept at $-20°$C until analysis. Total urine was collected every 6 h, the total volume was recorded, and a 20 ml aliquot was frozen until analysis.

The parent compound and its metabolite SN-38 were simultaneously assayed by high-performance liquid chromatography (HPLC) with fluorescence detection, as previously described.[27] Briefly, drug and metabolite concentrations were determined from peak area ratios of either compound to the internal standard (camptothecin) by reference to a calibration curve performed daily. This assay measures the total CPT-11 and SN-38, i.e., the hydrolized form is converted to the lactone form after acidification of biological samples.

Nonlinear regression analyses of CPT-11 plasma concentrations were performed with PC-NONLIN (Statistical Consultants, Inc., Lexington, Kentucky, U.S.A.). Pharmacokinetic parameters were determined using standard formulae.[28] Briefly, the half-lives were calculated as 0.693 divided by the corresponding elimination rate constant; the area under the plasma concentration versus time curve (AUC) was determined by the trapezoidal method with extrapolation to infinity; the volume of distribution at steady state (Vdss) was determined as $Vdss = Dose \times AUMC/AUC^2$, where AUMC is the area under the first moment curve that describes the time course of the plasma concentrations; the total plasma clearance (CL) was calculated as the Dose/AUC. The concentration at the end of i.v. infusion (Cmax) was the actual plasma concentration assayed. For the metabolite SN-38, the following parameters were determined: the maximum concentration achieved (Cmax), the AUC determined by the trapezoidal method, and the apparent elimination half-life.

III. RESULTS AND DISCUSSION

A. PATIENTS

The characteristics of the 152 patients entered so far in three Phase I studies are presented in Table 1. CPT-11 was administered as a 30-min IV infusion according to three different schedules: daily for three consecutive days every three weeks, weekly for three weeks, and once every three weeks.

B. PHARMACOKINETICS

As part of these Phase I studies, clinical pharmacokinetics of both CPT-11 and its active metabolite SN-38 were simultaneously determined at doses ranging from 33 to 400 mg/m^2. We report here the pharmacokinetics obtained on the first course only in 67 patients to prevent any possible influence of prior CPT-11 treatment on pharmacokinetics or toxicity.

In the Phase I study evaluating a daily administration for three days every three weeks, the maximum tolerated dose (MTD) was 115 mg/m^2. A representative CPT-11 pharmacokinetic profile is presented in Figure 1 at 100 $mg/m^2/d$, which is the Phase II recommended dose level for this schedule of administration.[23] In the weekly administration for three weeks, the MTD was 145 mg/m^2, and Phase II recommended doses are 100 $mg/m^2/$ wk in high-risk patients, and 115 $mg/m^2/wk$ for low-risk patients.[24] For the once every three-week schedule,[25] the MTD has not been reached thusfar but could be greater than 500 mg/m^2. A representative CPT-11 plasma profile at the 350 mg/m^2 dose level is presented in Figure 1.

CPT-11 plasma disposition curves were bi- or tri-phasic with a mean terminal half-life of 10 h. CPT-11 volume of distribution (Vdss) was large (140 L/m^2). Pharmacokinetics was linear with mean clearance values of 15 $L/h/m^2$.

Although the interpatient variability was important, the CPT-11 area under the plasma concentration versus time curves (AUC) increased proportionally to the CPT-11 dose within the dose range studied (Figure 2a). No drug accumulation was observed except in three patients receiving the drug daily for three consecutive days. There were no marked differences among CPT-11 schedules regarding pharmacokinetic parameters.[29]

CPT-11 long disposition half-life could be of therapeutic advantage for this S-phase specific drug, by allowing prolonged exposure time for tumor cells *in vivo*. CPT-11 terminal half-life appears shorter than that of camptothecin sodium salt, which was

Table 1 **Patient characteristics (n = 152)**

Median age (range)	55 (23–74)
Sex	71 women, 81 men
Performance status	
grade 0	46
grade 1	82
grade 2	24
Tumor type	
colorectal	46
head and neck	17
breast	11
lung	11
ovary	10
unknown primary	10
liver	7
pancreas	7
soft tissue sarcoma	7
kidney	6
cervix	4
melanoma	4
oesophagus	3
stomach	3
others	6
Prior treatment	
chemotherapy	134
surgery	120
radiotherapy	69
none	8

reported to have a terminal half-life of 17–40 h.[7] CPT-11 terminal half-life is longer, however, than that reported for topotecan[30] (see Chapters 9 and 10).

The determination of SN-38 pharmacokinetics is of prime importance, since this active metabolite is about 100- to 400-fold more potent than the parent drug.[31,32] Metabolite SN-38 plasma levels were about 100-fold lower than corresponding CPT-11 levels and followed an apparent elimination profile similar to the parent compound (Figure 1). CPT-11 prolonged disposition half-life is probably responsible for the maintenance of cytotoxic concentrations of SN-38 *in vivo*, by providing a sustained formation of this active metabolite. Exposure (AUC) to SN-38 appeared to increase with the CPT-11 dose, although the interpatient variability was important (Figures 1 and 2b). As a matter of fact, active metabolite SN-38 AUCs were better correlated to the parent compound AUCs than with CPT-11 dose (Figure 3).

In the once every three-week schedule, CPT-11 urinary excretion increased with dose. CPT-11 urinary excretion was 11% for the dose range 66–115 mg/m^2, whereas it increased to 38% for doses comprised between 260 and 450 mg/m^2. These data may indicate a saturation of excretion and/or metabolism of this compound. Metabolite SN-38 excretion was minimal and represented about 0.2% of the CPT-11 dose.

C. TOXICITIES

The main side effects observed with CPT-11 were nausea-vomiting, diarrhea, leukoneutropenia, anemia, alopecia, and fatigue. For these toxicities, a high interpatient variability was noted.

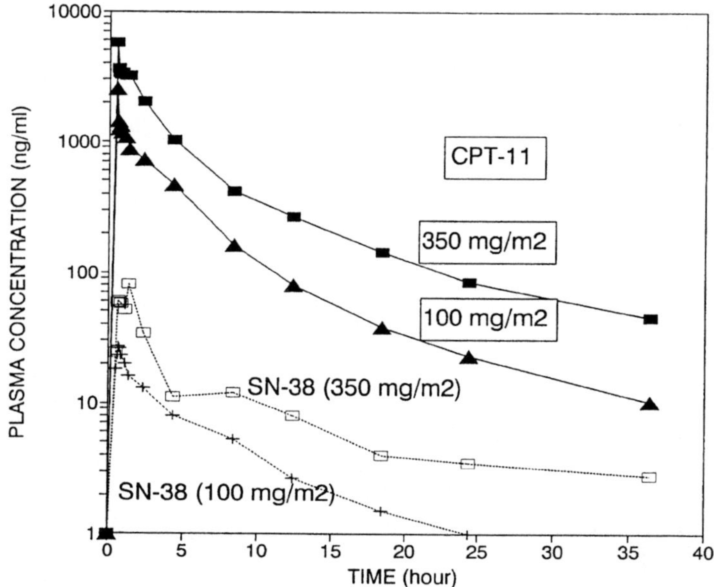

Figure 1 CPT-11 (solid lines) and active metabolite SN-38 (dashed lines) representative plasma profiles in two patients that received CPT-11 at 350 mg/m^2 and 100 mg/m^2, as a 30-min i.v. infusion. Solid squares, CPT-11 plasma levels at 350 mg/m^2; solid triangles, CPT-11 plasma levels at 100 mg/m^2; open squares, SN-38 plasma levels at CPT-11 dose of 350 mg/m^2; crosses, SN-38 plasma levels at CPT-11 dose of 100 mg/m^2.

The dose-limiting toxicities were leukoneutropenia and diarrhea in the daily × 3 schedule and in the weekly schedule. Leukoneutropenia appeared dose-related, non-cumulative, and reversible. For the once every three-week schedule, hematological toxicity may also be dose-limiting (based on presently available information). Diarrhea was less severe in the once every three-week schedule compared to the other schedules.

Schedule does not appear to influence markedly the toxicity of this agent for the daily × 3 and the weekly schedules, since approximately the same total dose could be administered, using these schemes of administration (e.g., a total dose of about 300–345 mg/m^2). These clinical observations are in agreement with preclinical data in tumor-bearing mice that showed that CPT-11 is also not markedly schedule-dependent.[13,14] As noted above, however, schedule appears to influence the severity of diarrhea, since it was less severe in the once every three-week schedule compared to other schedules.

D. RESPONSES

Although the optimal CPT-11 schedule and dose are not obviously defined in Phase I studies, partial responses were nevertheless observed in all three Phase I trials. Hints of antitumor activity were mainly noted in colorectal, cervical, and mammary tumors.[23-25]

CPT-11 anticancer activity observed in these Phase I trials is noteworthy, considering that optimal schedule and dose are not yet precisely defined for this compound. These observations confirm and extend the promising CPT-11 anticancer activity already observed at other institutions[18-22] (see also Chapters 6 and 7). The ongoing French Phase II trials will better identify the precise anticancer activity spectrum of this compound.

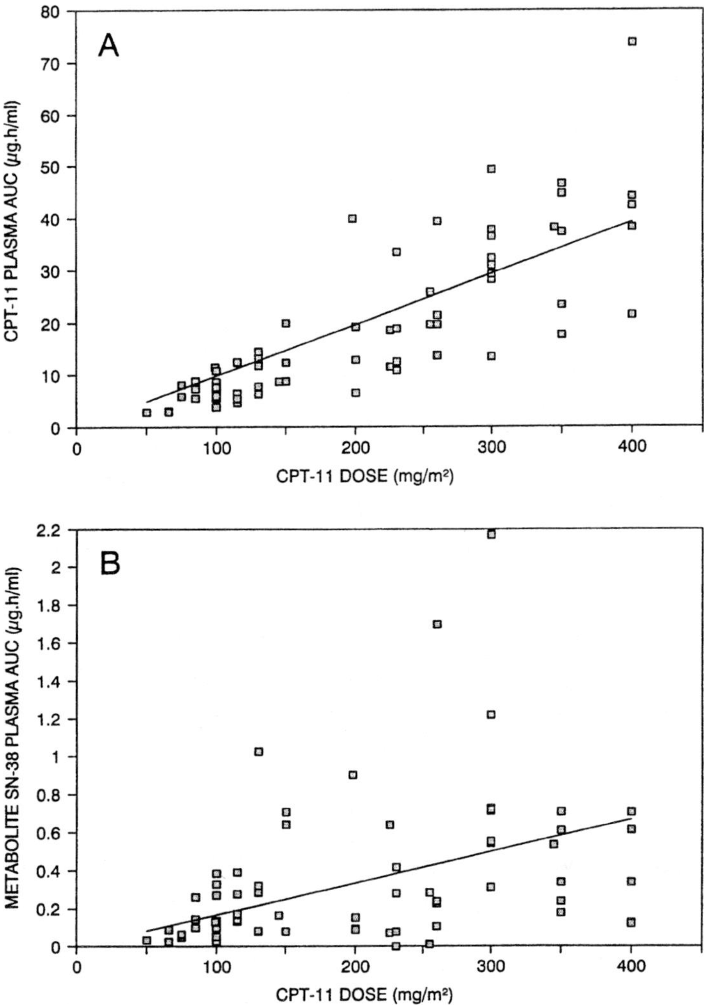

Figure 2 (A) CPT-11 area under the plasma concentration versus time curves (AUC) as a function of CPT-11 dose (r = 0.82, *p* < 0.001). (B) Active metabolite SN-38 AUC as a function of CPT-11 dose (r = 0.36, *p* < 0.01).

E. PHARMACOKINETIC-PHARMACODYNAMIC RELATIONSHIPS

In an attempt to define early pharmacokinetic-pharmacodynamic relationships that may be useful for further clinical testing of CPT-11, the pharmacokinetic parameters were tentatively correlated with the intensity of the main toxicities encountered with this drug. Since AUC usually correlates better with the pharmacological action of anticancer drugs, this pharmacokinetic parameter was chosen for correlation studies.

Although interpatient variability was important (Figure 4), CPT-11 AUC correlated significantly with the percent decrease in white blood cells. CPT-11 AUC also correlated significantly with the intensity of diarrhea in the weekly schedule.

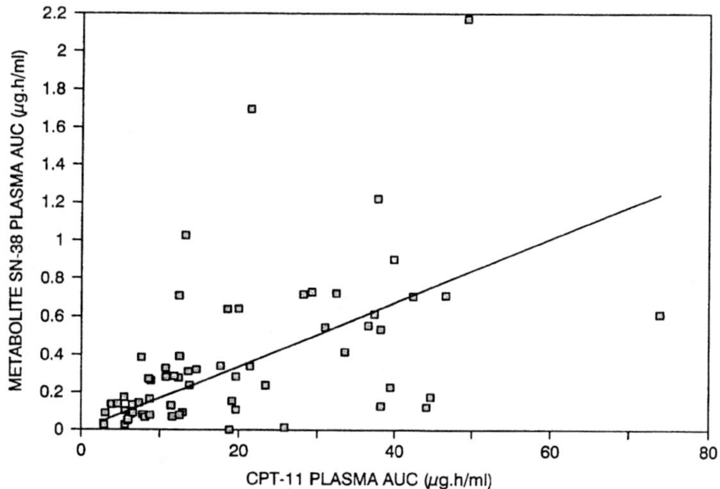

Figure 3 Active metabolite SN-38 area under the plasma concentration versus times curves (AUC) as a function of CPT-11 AUCs (r = 0.52, $p < 0.001$).

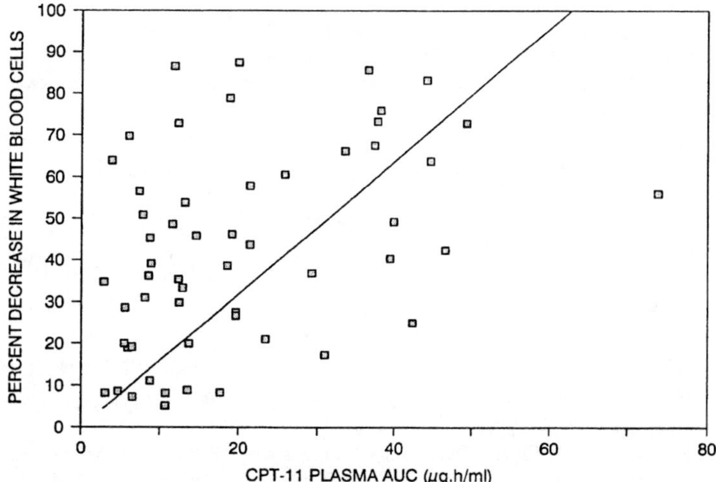

Figure 4 Percent decrease in white blood cells at nadir, as a function of CPT-11 dose (r = 0.39, $p < 0.01$).

Active metabolite SN-38 AUC was also significantly correlated with percent decrease in white blood cells. In the weekly schedule, SN-38 AUC was also significantly correlated with the intensity of diarrhea.

Although responses were noted in the three Phase I trials, the relatively small number of responders preclude any meaningful correlation analysis with pharmacokinetics for the moment. Responses were, however, observed at the highest doses administered in each Phase I trial. Ongoing Phase II trials will undoubtedly define better the relationships between CPT-11 and/or SN-38 pharmacokinetics and anticancer activity.

IV. SUMMARY

The data presented herein indicate that pharmacokinetics could be valuable for predicting the intensity of both diarrhea and leukoneutropenia, which are CPT-11 dose-limiting toxicities. Ongoing Phase II trials will hopefully uncover other pharmacokinetic-pharmacodynamic relationships, especially with regard to anticancer efficacy, that could be useful in the clinical management of this interesting anticancer drug.

ACKNOWLEDGMENTS

We are grateful to M. Ré, M. Guiguin, and I. Barilero for their skillful laboratory assistance. We also thank the following organizations that made these studies possible: the Laboratoire Roger Bellon, the Institut National de la Santé et de la Recherche Médicale (INSERM), the Centre National de la Recherche Scientifique (CNRS), and the Association pour la Recherche sur le Cancer.

REFERENCES

1. **Wall, M. E., Wani, M. C., Cook, C. E., Palmar, K. H., McPhail, A. T., and Sim, G. A.,** Plant antitumor agents. I. The isolation and structure of camptothecin, a novel alkaloidal leukemia and antitumor inhibitor from *Camptotheca acuminata. J. Am. Chem. Soc.*, 88, 3888, 1966.
2. **Li, L. H., Fraser, T. J., Olin, E. J., and Bhuyan, B. K.,** Action of camptothecin on mammalian cells in culture. *Cancer Res.*, 32, 2643, 1972.
3. **Drewinko, G., Freireich, E. J., and Gottlied, J. A.,** Lethal activity of camptothecin sodium on human lymphoma cells. *Cancer Res.*, 34, 747, 1974.
4. **Gallo, R. C., Whang-Peng, J., and Adamson, R. H.,** Studies on the antitumor activity, mechanism of action, and cell cycle effects of camptothecin. *J. Natl. Cancer Inst.*, 46, 789, 1971.
5. **Moertel, C. G., Shutt, A. J., Reitemeier, R. J., and Hahn, R. G.,** Phase II study of camptothecin (NSC 100880) in the treatment of advanced gastrointestinal cancer. *Cancer Chemother. Rep.*, 56, 95, 1972.
6. **Gottlieb, J. A. and Luce, J. K.,** Treatment of malignant melanoma with camptothecin (NSC 100880). *Cancer Chemother. Rep.*, 56, 103, 1972.
7. **Gottlieb, J. A., Guarino, A. M., Call, J. B., Oliverio, V. T., and Block, J. B.,** Preliminary pharmacologic and clinical evaluation of camptothecin sodium (NSC 100880). *Cancer Chemother. Rep.*, 54, 461, 1970.
8. **Muggia, F. M., Creaven, P. J., Hansen, H. H., and Selawry, O. S.,** Phase I clinical trials of weekly and daily treatment with camptothecin (NSC 100880). Correlation with clinical studies. *Cancer Chemother. Rep.*, 56, 515, 1972.
9. **Shaeppi, V., Fleischman, R. W., and Cooney, D. A.,** Toxicity of camptothecin (NSC 100880). *Cancer Chemother. Rep.*, 58, 25, 1974.
10. **Kunimoto, T., Nitta, K., Tanaka, T., Uehara, N., Baba, H., Takeuchi, M., Yokokura, T., Sawada, S., Miyasaka T., and Mutai, M.,** Antitumor activity of 7-ethyl-10-[4-(1-piperidino] carbonyloxy-camptothecin, a novel water-soluble derivative of camptothecin, against murine tumors. *Cancer Res.*, 47, 5944, 1987.
11. **Matsuzaki, T., Yokokura, T., Mutai M., and Tsuruo, T.,** Inhibition of spontaneous and experimental mestatasis by a new derivation of camptothecin, CPT-11, in mice. *Cancer Chemother. Pharmacol.*, 21, 308, 1988.
12. **Tsuruo, T., Matsuzaki, T., Matsushita, M., Saito, H., and Yokokura, T.,** Antitumor effect of CPT-11, a new derivative of camptothecin, against pleiotropic drug-resistant tumors *in vitro* and *in vivo. Cancer Chemother. Pharmacol.*, 21, 71, 1988.

13. **Bissery, M. C., Mathieu-Boué, A., and Lavelle, F.,** Experimental antitumor activity of CPT-11 *in vitro* and *in vivo. Annals of Oncology*, 3, Suppl. 1, 82, Abstract 93, 1992.

14. **Bissery, M. C., Mathieu-Boué, A., and Lavelle, F.,** Preclinical evaluation of CPT-11, a camptothecin derivative. *Proc. Amer. Assoc. Cancer Res.*, 32, 402, abstract 2389, 1991.

15. **Hsiang, Y. H., Hertzberg, R., Hecht, S., and Liu, L. F.,** Camptothecin induces protein-linked DNA breaks via mammalian DNA topoisomerase I. *J. Biol. Chem.*, 260, 14873, 1985.

16. **Covey, J. M., Jaxel, C., Kohn, K. W., and Pommier, Y.,** Protein-linked DNA strand breaks induced in mammalian cells by camptothecin, an inhibitor of topoisomerase I. *Cancer Res.*, 49, 5016, 1989.

17. **Shugimoto, Y., Tsukahara, S., Oh-hara, T., Isoe, T., and Tsuruo, T.,** Decreased expression of DNA topoisomerase I in camptothecin-resistant tumor cell lines as determined by a monoclonal antibody. *Cancer Res.*, 50, 6925, 1990.

18. **Tagushi, T., Wakui, A., and Hasegawa, K.,** Phase I clinical study of CPT-11. Research Group of CPT-11. *Gan-to-Kagakuryoho*, 17, 115, 1990.

19. **Fukuoka, M., Nitani, H., Suzuki, A., Motomiya, M., Hasegawa, K., Nishiwaki, Y., Kuriyama, T., Ariyoshi, Y., Negoro, S., Masuda, N., Nakajima, S., and Taguchi, T.,** for the CPT-11 Lung Cancer Study Group, A phase II study of CPT-11, a new derivative of camptothecin, for previously untreated non-small cell lung cancer. *J. Clin. Oncol.*, 10, 16, 1992.

20. **Ohno, R., Okada, K., Masaoka, T., Kuramoto, A., Arima, T., Yoshido, Y., Ariyoshi, H., Ichimaru, M., Sakai, Y., Oguro, M., Ito, Y., Morishima, Y., Yokomaku, S., and Ota, K.,** An early phase II study of CPT-11: a new derivative of camptothecin for the treatment of leukemia and lymphoma. *J. Clin. Oncol.*, 8, 1907, 1990.

21. **Masuda, N., Fukuoka, M., Kusunoki, Y., Matsui, K., Takifuji, N., Kudoh, S., Negoro, S., Nishioka, M., Nakagawa, K., and Takada, M.,** CPT-11 : A new derivative of camptothecin for the treatment of refractory or relapsed small cell lung cancer. *J. Clin. Oncol.*, 10, 1225, 1992.

22. **Shimada, Y., Yoshino, M., Wakui, A., Nakao, I., Futatsuki, K., Sakata, Y., Kambe, M., Taguchi, T., and CPT-11 Gastrointestinal Cancer Study Group,** Phase II study of CPT-11, a new camptothecin derivative, in the patients with metastatic colorectal cancer. *Proc. Am. Soc. Clin. Oncol.*, 10, 135, abstract 408, 1991.

23. **Clavel, M., Mathieu-Boué, A., Dumortier, A., Chabot, G. G., Cote, C., Bissery, M. C., and Marty, M.,** Phase I study of CPT-11 administered as a daily infusion for 3 consecutive days. *Proc. Amer. Assoc. Cancer Res.*, 33, 262, abstract 1568, 1992.

24. **Culine, S., de Forni, M., Extra, J. M., Chabot, G. G., Madelaine, I., Hérait, P., Bugat, R., Marty, M., and Mathieu-Boué, A.,** Phase I study of the camptothecin analogue CPT-11, using a weekly schedule. *Proc. Amer. Soc. Clin. Oncol.*, 11, 110, abstract 263, 1992.

25. **Gandia, D., Armand, J. P., Chabot, G. G., Abigerges, D., Rougier, P., Ruffié, P., Cote, C., and Mathieu-Boué, A.,** Phase I study of the new camptothecin analogue CPT-11 administered every 3 weeks. *Proc. Amer. Assoc. Cancer Res.*, 33, 260, abstract 1560, 1992.

26. **Miller, A. B., Hoogstraten, B., and Staquet, M.,** Reporting results of cancer treatment. *Cancer*, 47, 207, 1981.

27. **Barilero, I., Gandia, D., Armand, J. P., Mathieu-Boué, A., Ré, M., Gouyette, A., and Chabot, G. G.,** Simultaneous determination of the camptothecin analogue CPT-11 and its active metabolite SN-38 by high-performance liquid chromatography: application to plasma pharmacokinetic studies in cancer patients. *J. Chromatogr. (Biomed. Appl.)*, 575, 275, 1992.

28. **Gibaldi, M. and Perrier, D.,** *Pharmacokinetics.* Second edition, Marcel Dekker, Inc., New York and Basel, 1982, 494 pages.
29. **Chabot, G. G., Abigerges, D., Gandia, D., Armand, J. P., Clavel, M., de Forni, M., Suc, E., Bugat, R., Culine, S., Extra, J. M., Marty, M., Mathieu-Boué, A., and Gouyette, A.,** Pharmacokinetic-pharmacodynamic relationships in patients administered with CPT-11, a new camptothecin analogue. *Proc. Amer. Assoc. Cancer Res.,* 33, 266, abstract 1596, 1992.
30. **Wall, J., Burris, H., Rodriguez, G., Brown, T., Weiss, G., Kuhn, J., Brown, J., Johnson, R., Friedman, C., Mann, W., and Von Hoff, D.,** Phase I trial of topotecan (SKF 104864) in patients with refractory solid tumors. *Proc. Amer. Soc. Clin. Oncol.,* 10, 98, abstract 261, 1992.
31. **Kaneda, N., Nagata, H., Furuta, T., and Yokokura, T.,** Metabolism and pharmacokinetics of the camptothecin analogue CPT-11 in the mouse. *Cancer Res.,* 50, 1715, 1990.
32. **Kaneda, N. and Yokokura, T.,** Nonlinear pharmacokinetics of CPT-11 in rats. *Cancer Res.,* 30, 1721, 1990.

Topotecan Clinical Trials in the United States

Howard S. Hochster

CONTENTS

I. INTRODUCTION

Topotecan (NSC-603071), 20(*S*)-9-dimethylaminomethyl-10-hydroxy-camptothecin, is a semisynthetic analog of the plant alkaloid, camptothecin. This compound was designed to overcome many of the problems associated with the sodium salt of the parent compound, based on the following preclinical rationale:

1. Camptothecin acts by inhibition of the nuclear enzyme topoisomerase-1.
2. The lactone form is the active moiety of the compound.
3. The sodium salt has 10-fold less antitumor activity than the lactone.
4. Structure-function relationships clearly demonstrate that A-ring substitution (at the 9 and 10 positions) increases activity.
5. Substitution with polar groups increases the aqueous solubility of the lactone form.

With this preclinical rationale in mind, investigators at SmithKline Beecham synthesized a family of camptothecin analogs, including topotecan. This latter compound has shown remarkable preclinical activity, has recently completed Phase I testing, and is in broad Phase II testing at this time.

A. BACKGROUND

Camptothecin (Figure 1) is the natural product derived as an extract of the Chinese plant *Camptotheca acuminata*. It was first discovered to have antitumor activity by NCI investigators.[1] The development of camptothecin and its analogs is discussed elsewhere in this volume.

Following early clinical trials of camptothecin sodium salt[2-3] (and see Chapter 3 in this book), the drug remained of little interest, as it was considered to be minimally active and

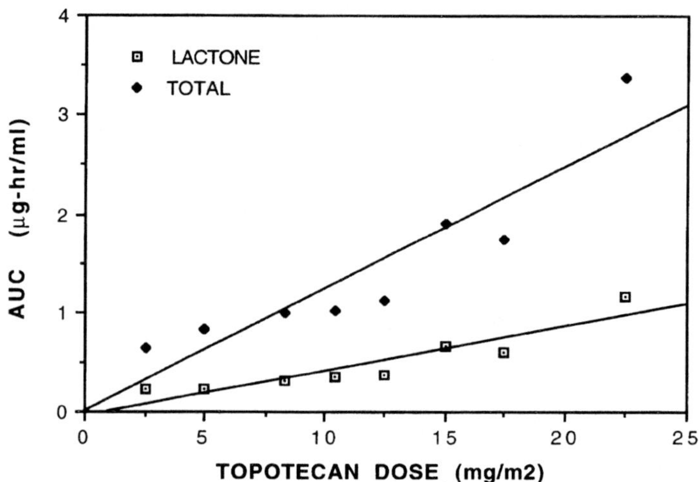

Figure 1   AUC as a function of topotecan dose given over 30 minutes.[20]

to have unpredictable toxicity. Whether oral administration of camptothecin, as the lactone form, will have similar toxicities remains to be established (see Chapter 5 in this book). Following the early trials, interest in this family of compounds waned. Later, important preclinical investigations rekindled interest in this group of compounds through the greater understanding of their mechanism of action.

Liu and co-workers, as part of a drug development group, investigated activity of certain topoisomerase-2 inhibitory drugs. Since camptothecin shared many common properties with topoisomerase-2 inhibitors (such as cell-cycle specificity and induction of protein-associated DNA breaks), this drug was tested in an assay for topoisomerase-2 activity that happened to use topoisomerase-1 as a co-factor. From these experiments, it became quite clear that camptothecin acted through inhibition of topoisomerase-1.[4-5] Once this mechanism of action was discovered, many other camptothecin analogs were synthesized and studied for their activity as topoisomerase-1 inhibitors.[6-8] These structure-function studies clearly demonstrate that (1) the five-member ring is necessary for inhibition of topoisomerase-1; (2) an S-configuration at the C-20 chiral center is necessary for activity; (3) ring opening of the lactone, producing the carboxylate form, results in approximately one-tenth the activity of the lactone; (4) substitution in the A ring at the 9, 10 and 11 positions tends to increase binding to topoisomerase-1 and *in vitro* activity; while (5) substitution at the 12 position seems to interfere with binding to enzyme and decrease activity.

Based on these considerations, Johnson and collaborators at SmithKline Beecham postulated that they could produce an analog of camptothecin which would avoid the problems of poor aqueous solubility and avid protein binding of the parent compound.[9-10] Production of a water-soluble lactone analog which would be active *per se* as opposed to the sodium salt (which requires relactonization to be active) was achieved by substitution in the 9 position by the amino alkyl family of constituents.[11] The 10-hydroxy substitution also increases water solubility and reduces plasma protein binding. *In vitro* testing showed that this camptothecin analog is equivalent to that of the parent compound in terms of inhibition of topoisomerase-1, while producing a slightly higher IC_{50} for L1210 leukemia cells. Nonetheless, topotecan produced a 173% increase in life span of mice bearing L1210 leukemia compared to 118% for camptothecin.[11] Because of the favorable preclinical characteristics of this 10-hydroxy, 9-dimethylaminomethyl-substituted camptothecin, topotecan was selected for further testing.

II. RESULTS AND DISCUSSION

A. PRECLINICAL ACTIVITY

1. Pharmacology

Topotecan was tested in several *in vitro* systems showing its effect on topoisomerase-1.[12] *In vitro* testing clearly demonstrated that the drug activity is mediated by this enzyme, since it has no activity in topoisomerase-1 lacking yeast cell mutants. Furthermore, neither topotecan nor camptothecin bind to isolated DNA and therefore have no direct effect. On the other hand, when combined with cells or isolated nuclei, topotecan produced nearly 100% protein-associated single-strand DNA breaks, while camptothecin was less efficient. With both compounds, protein-associated breaks rapidly reversed within 15–30 minutes following removal of the compound.

2. *In Vivo* Activity

Topotecan has demonstrated a high degree of activity in a wide range of animal tumor models including xenografts with HT29 human colon cancer and murine tumors including colon 26, 38, and 51; Madison and Lewis Lung carcinomas; M5076 reticulum cell sarcoma; mammary adenocarcinoma 16-C; and P388 and L1210 leukemia.

In xenograft experiments with HT29 colon cancer, i.v. topotecan was active against subcutaneously implanted tumor, resulting in growth delay of 18–24 days. This is a remarkable result in a xenograft known to be particularly refractory to established chemotherapeutic agents.

The B16 melanoma studies involved mice with tumors implanted subcutaneously (s.c.); intraperitoneally (i.p.), or intravenously (i.v.) and treatment either intravenously or intraperitoneally. In each case, topotecan significant delayed tumor growth and increased survival by 45–95%. Of note for the i.v.-implanted tumors treated four times per day at three-hour intervals once a week for two weeks, 50% of mice treated intraperitoneally or orally were long-term survivors (> 90 days). Multi-fractionated dosing seemed to have greater effect against these tumors. In ADJ-BC6 plasmacytoma, similar results were seen including 100% growth inhibition at the MTD (15 mg/kg), though no cures were seen.

Using subcutaneous Lewis lung carcinoma, topotecan produced an increased life span of 200% compared to nontreated controls, an effect equal to cisplatin. Similar activity was seen with oral administration. For i.v.-implanted tumors with i.v. administration, increased life span was $\geq$ 200%, with 11/14 mice being long-term survivors. In the case of Madison lung carcinoma, however, topotecan was no more effective than either cyclophosphamide or cisplatin causing only a marginal increase in life span of no therapeutic significance. Topotecan (i.p.) against subcutaneously implanted mammary adenocarcinoma 16C showed a 73% growth inhibition, which was comparable to cisplatin (3 mg/kg). Somewhat better results were seen with increasing dose, yielding 96% growth inhibition, but no long-term survivors.

For the murine colon carcinomas 26, 38, and 51, topotecan was evaluated in intraperitoneal or subcutaneously implanted tumors. Topotecan was administered i.p. or i.v. and compared to cisplatinum controls. In all three murine colon carcinomas, topotecan was found to be effective and had activity comparable to cisplatin. The activity was maximized when the drug was given by a split-dose regimen. Similar results were also seen with P388 and L1210 leukemias, though one study with intracranial tumor administration suggested that topotecan was less effective in crossing the blood-brain barrier than BCNU. Of particular note were i.v. single or divided dose regimens for leukemia yielded curative activity, especially with the split dosing which gave the longest drug exposure. In general, tumor burden was decreased by 4–7 logs, and life span was prolonged from 170–250%.

Table 1 Cancers with shown topotecan activity in phase I studies

NSCLC	(6)
OVARIAN	(5)
COLORECTAL	(2)

Note: NSCLC, non-small cell lung cancer.

Table 2 High dose topotecan in leukemia

Institution	Schedule	MTD (mg/m2)	Response
JHOC	5d CIV q3w–4w	—	—
MDA	5d CIV q3–4w	10.0 mg/m2 × 5	3 CR/2PR

Note: JHOC = Johns Hopkins Oncology Center; MDA = MD Anderson Hospital.

B. CLINICAL TRIALS

Phase I clinical trials with topotecan have been conducted under sponsorship of SmithKline and the NCI utilizing several schedules including daily × 5 (over 30 minutes, as a short infusion or "bolus"), 30-minute infusion every three weeks, 24-hour infusion every three weeks, 24-hour infusion weekly, 120-hr infusion every three weeks (later reduced to 72 hours), and prolonged 21-day infusion. As of December 1, 1993, more than 300 patients had been enrolled in Phase I studies. Results of these studies are reported in Table 3. In general, the major toxicity seen in these programs has been myelosuppression or thrombocytopenia. Some diarrhea, nausea, and vomiting has been seen in these heavily pretreated patients, and alopecia has been reported occasionally. Two groups have particularly studied the issue of cumulative myelosuppression and have reported that topotecan, even when given up to 10 cycles, did not appear to produce evidence of cumulative bone marrow toxicity.[15]

The daily × 5 schedule has been reproduced in two different institutions.[13-16] In both instances, the MTD was found to be 1.5–2.0 mg/m^2/d depending upon the degree of prior therapy. Also in both cases, dose could not be escalated with G-CSF due to Grade 3–4 thrombocytopenia despite protection against neutropenia. Dose intensity for these regimens is approximately 2.5–3.0 mg/m^2/wk. Two institutions have performed studies of 24-hour continuous infusion given every three weeks,[17-19] while the Fox Chase group studied topotecan by 24-hour infusion weekly.[20-21] The reported MTD for the three-week schedule is 5–10 mg/m^2, producing a dose intensity of 2–3 mg/m^2/wk with neutropenia being dose-limiting toxicity. The Fox Chase Program suggested that this drug could be given at 2 mg/m^2/weekly for up to three weeks for a dose intensity of 1.5 mg/m^2/wk. All these regimens produce similar dose intensity, without any great advantage for a particular schedule.

1. Longer Infusions

Infusional schedules are of particular interest with this drug since the cell cycle specificity suggests that prolonged administration may produce greater effects. This has been documented in murine tumor models showing improvement in activity with a split-dosing schedule. Further studies with other camptothecin analogs showed that administration over many weeks can be safely given while curing mice of human tumors xenografts.[26]

Table 3 Adult topotecan phase I studies

Institution	Schedule	MTD (mg/m²)	Dose Intensity (mg/m²/wk)	Ref.
Johns Hopkins	d × 5 q3w (30 min inf) PLUS G-CSF d6	1.5–2.0 × 5 same	2.5–3.3	13–15
MSKCC	d × 5 q3w (30 min inf) PLUS G-CSF	1.25–1.5 × 5 1.5 × 5	2.5–2.92	16
MD Anderson	24 hr CIV q3w	10	3.3	17–18
Mayo Clinics	24 hr CIV q3w	5.0	1.7	19
Fox Chase	24 hr CIV qwk	2.0	1.5	20–21
UTSA	5d CIV q3w	0.68 × 5	1.2	22–23
	3d CIV q3w	1.60 × 3	1.6	—
CWRU	3d CIV q week × 4	0.66 × 3	1.98	—
NYU	low dose CIV × 7–21d	0.53 × 21	2.8	25

Note: MSKCC = Memorial Sloan Kettering Cancer Center; UTSA = University of Texas at San Antonio; CWRU = Case Western Reserve University; NYU = New York University Medical Center.

A five-day infusion was carried out at the University of Texas at San Antonio, which resulted in a disappointingly low dose intensity, with an MTD of 0.68 mg/m²/day × 5 days consecutively.[22-23] Dose-limiting toxicity was thrombocytopenia. Because of the low-dose intensity (1.2 mg/m²/wk) using the five-day infusion, the duration of the infusion was shortened to three days (72-hour infusion every three weeks) with an MTD of 1.60 mg/m²/d.

2. 21-Day Continuous Infusion

Clinical trials using the most prolonged infusion schedule have been conducted by the group at the New York University Medical Center, where the drug has safely been given up to 21 days.[22-23] Initial dosing was at 0.2 mg/m²/d for seven days, but later was safely extended to 0.7 mg/m²/d for 21 days using ambulatory infusion pumps. At this highest dose, three of four heavily pretreated patients developed Grade 4 thrombocytopenia. The recommended dose for Phase II studies was determined to be the prior dose level, 0.53 mg/m²/d which produces a dose intensity of 2.8 mg/m²/wk. This exceeds the dose intensity of the recommended Phase II daily × 5 schedule (dose intensity of 1.9 mg/m²/wk) by nearly 50%. Dose-limiting toxicity for this schedule, like the other schedules, has been myelosuppression, with more severe thrombocytopenia than neutropenia as seen with the bolus schedules. Most patients receiving multiple cycles also required red cell transfusions. Nonhematologic toxicity associated with this regimen has been quite mild, consisting mainly of Grade 1–2 fatigue. Minimal alopecia was seen and infectious complications, despite prolonged intravenous administration, were minimal. Further testing of this schedule is now continuing for minimally pre-treated patients at a dose of 0.6 mg/m²/d × 21 days and for chemotherapy-naive patients a dose of 0.7 mg/m²/d × 21 days has been tolerated well in several patients. The dose intensity for this level is nearly 3.7 mg/m²/wk.

To date, responses were seen in this trial in patients with renal cancer and non-small cell lung cancer. More importantly, measurable partial remissions were seen in heavily treated patients with ovarian cancer (three of six treated) and breast cancer (one of two patients treated). This response rate of 50% in a small number of heavily pretreated ovarian cancer patients is particularly exciting in view of the 15% response rate reported by investigators at MD Anderson using the daily × 5 schedule.

Table 4 Topotecan pharmacokinetic studies*

Institution	Dose/Schedule (mg/m²)	C_{peak} (ng/ml)	C_{ss} (ng/ml)	$t_{1/2}\beta$ (h)	CL_{tb} (l/hr/m²)	Vd_{ss} (l/m²)	Ref.
JHOC	0.5 × 5	9.4		3.0 ± 0.31	77.6 ± 14.5	25.6 ± 3.8	13–15
	2.5	23.2					
UTSA	30 min infusion						
	2.5	130		3.4 ± 1.1	25.7 ± 6.7	76.4 ± 18.5	22–23
	22.5	581					
UTSA	1.3/d × 3 d		4				22–23
FCCC	1.5/d × 24 h		7.0 ± 1.8	4.9	10.8 ± 2.2	61 ± 19	20–21
NCI (peds)	2.0/d × 24 h		2.9	2.4	26.5 ± 8.7		31
	3.0		5.3				
	4.0		9.2				
	5.5		9.6				
	7.5		14.1				
NYU	0.53/d × 21 d		3.9 ± 1.5				25
	0.70/d × 21 d		5.1 ± 1.2				

*All values are for the lactone species.

Note: JHOC = Johns Hopkins Oncology Center; UTSA = University of Texas at San Antonio; FCCC = Fox Chase Cancer Center; NCI = National Cancer Institute; NYU = New York University Medical Center.

3. Objective Responses

Despite treating a typical Phase I patient population, with moderate to heavy pretreatment, clinical antitumor responses were reported on most schedules, including the daily × 5, weekly 24-h infusion, and 21-day infusion. Several responses were reported in patients with non-small cell lung cancer and with ovarian cancer. Two patients with colon cancer also responded. Due to small numbers of patients and the general mixture of tumor types, it is impossible to recommend one schedule over another based on activity. It is clear, however, that these tumor types are of great interest for Phase II testing and are likely to be responsive to topotecan.

4. Phase II Studies

Studies in a broad spectrum of disease have been planned for Phase II testing of topotecan under NCI auspices. Table 5 lists approved protocols by CTEP and their current status. All studies are to be performed on a daily × 5 schedule. SmithKline Beecham is also conducting several Phase II studies (Table 6), all to be performed at a dose and schedule of 1.5 mg/m² daily × 5. These studies are now underway, and the ovarian cancer study has been reported with a response rate of 15% in previously treated patients. A somewhat different approach has been adopted for the treatment of refractory Acute Non-lymphocytic Leukemia (ANLL). Phase II studies at Johns Hopkins Oncology Center and MD Anderson Cancer Center are being conducted using higher doses of Topotecan as a 5-day continuous infusion. The study at MD Anderson has reached an MTD of 2.0 mg/m²/d with dose-limiting mucositis at the dose of 11.8 mg/m²/course. Three patients who were heavily pretreated for ANLL had complete remissions, while two had partial remissions. Overall response rate with 19% in AML and 24% in AUL.[25] The JHOC study has not progressed as far, though several patients have had cytoreductive responses. *In vitro* studies have also suggested synergistic cytotoxicity between topotecan and various other chemotherapeutic agents. Several clinical trials based on these preclinical data have been

Table 5 **Phase II topotecan studies — NCI sponsored**

Disease	Institution	Schedule $(mg/m^2/d) \times 5$
Breast	URoch	1.5 q3w
Esoph/gastric	NYU	2.0 q4w
Gastric	SWOG 9150	1.5 q3w
	MSKCC	1.5 q3w + G-CSF
Head & neck	UAB	1.5 q3w
Hepatoma	SWOG 9151	1.5 q3w
Leukemia (CLL)	MDA	1.5 q3–4w
NSCLC	DFCI	2.0 q3w
SCLC	MDA	1.25 q3w
Lymphoma	OSU	1.25 q3w
Melanoma	OSU	1.5 q3w
Ovarian	JHOC	1.5 q 3 w
Pancreas	Fox Chase	1.5 q3w
	JHOC	1.5 q3w
Prostate	Fox Chase	1.5 q4w
Renal	MSKCC	1.5 q4w
Renal/melanoma	BRMP	1.5 q3w+GM-CSF
Sarcoma	NCIC	1.5 q3w

Note: URoch = University of Rochester; NYU = New York University Medical Center; SWOG = Southwest Oncology Group; MSKCC = Memorial Sloan Kettering Cancer Center; UAB = University of Alabama; MDA = MD Anderson Hospital; DFCI = Dana Farber Cancer Institute; OSU = Ohio State University; JHOC = Johns Hopkins Oncology Center; NCIC = National Cancer Institute of Canada.

Table 6 **Topotecan phase II studies SmithKline Beecham sponsored**

Disease	Schedule $(mg/m^2/d) \times 5$ Bolus
Breast	$1.5 \times 5d$
Colon	$1.5 \times 5d$
NSCLC	$1.5 \times 5d$
SCLC	$1.5 \times 5d$
Ovarian	$1.5 \times 5d$

approved and have begun combining topotecan with cisplatin, etoposide, and taxol (Table 7). These studies will, in some cases, look at the sequence of drug administration and the use of the growth factor, G-CSF.

C. PHARMACOLOGY

Phase I studies to date have investigated pharmacokinetics of topotecan. It is important to note that two species of topotecan can be determined using HPLC with fluorescent

Table 7 Topotecan combination trials

Institution	Schedule	Dose (mg/m^2)
CALGB	30 min IV d $\times$ 5 q3w	1.0 $\times$ 5
	CDDP 1 h IV q3w	25 (escalating)
UTSA	3d CIV	0.17 $\times$ 3 (escalating)
	VP-16	100 mg/m^2/d IV d7-9
JHOC	IV d $\times$ 5 q3w	0.75 $\times$ 5
	CDDP IV d1 or d5 q3w	50
	G-CSF	
GOG	Topotecan d $\times$ 5 q4w	0.75 $\times$ 5
	Taxol 24 h CIV	135
	G-CSF	

Note: CALGB = Cancer and Leukemia Group B; UTSA = University of Texas at San Antonio; JHOC = Johns Hopkins Oncology Center; GOG = Gynecologic Oncology Group.

detection: the intact lactone form and the "open-ring" carboxylate form, which exist in equilibrium in solution and in physiologic fluids. In order to preserve the ratio of the open and closed forms accurately, cold methanol is immediately added to the rapidly separated plasma in one commonly used method.[28] This procedure deproteinates the plasma and "stop-freezes" the open and closed forms at the existing ratio. Half the sample is analyzed to determine the amount of lactone using a calibrated standard curve. Then the other half of the sample is acidified, typically with phosphoric acid, to convert all remaining carboxylate into the lactone form and to determine chromatographically the total amount of drug.

The San Antonio group studied topotecan 30-minute infusion (bolus schedule) every three weeks began at a dose of 2.5 mg/m^2 and escalated to 22.5 mg/m^2.[29-30] Dose-limiting toxicity was neutropenia. In the patients studied for pharmacokinetics, the data for blood levels of the lactone fit a two-compartment model with beta half-life of 3.4 $\pm$ 1.1 hours. For total drug with figure was 4.3 $\pm$ 1.8 hours. Clearance was 4.8 $\pm$ 0.9 l/h/m^2 with steady state Vd of 76.4 $\pm$ 18.5 l/m^2. AUC for both lactone and total drug was linear in proportion to dose (Figure 1). The ratio of AUC for lactone:total drug was 0.33 $\pm$ .04 across all dose levels.

Other studies of topotecan pharmacokinetics using bolus schedule (daily $\times$ 5) were carried out by the group at Johns Hopkins.[10] They found a similar beta half-life for the lactone of 3.0 $\pm$ 0.3 hours, but somewhat higher clearance of 77.6 $\pm$ 14.5 l/hr/m^2. AUC was linear but showed considerable individual overlap. For the highest dose level (2.5 mg/m^2), the peak concentration was 23.2 ng/ml (range 11.6 to 43.9). While percent decrease in ANC (neutrophil count) at the nadir correlated with dose administered in a sigmoidal (Emax) model, there was no correlation with AUC for the lactone.

The NCI pediatric study[31] (see Table 8) confirmed these values in children, on a 24-hour infusion schedule. Steady-state concentration ranged from 2.9 ng/ml for 2.0 mg/m^2 (over 24 hours) to 14.1 ng/ml for the highest dose (7.5 mg/m^2). Again Css was linear and beta half-life was similar to other reports at 2.4 h.

An adult study of weekly 24-hour infusion[19-20] at the MTD of 1.5 mg/m^2 weekly showed a Css of 7.0 $\pm$ 1.8 ng/ml with a somewhat faster clearance than other reports, 10.8 $\pm$ 2.2 l/h/m^2. Beta half-life was slightly longer than other reports at 4.9 h. At NYU we have determined the steady-state levels in those treated at dose levels of 0.4 mg/m^2/d or greater, where drug levels were detectable using an improved assay for determination of very low drug levels.[25] In this group of patients, 58 determinations were made in 15 patients. Figure 2 shows the mean steady-state concentration for lactone and total drug at each dose level.

Table 8 Pediatric topotecan trials

Institution	Schedule	MTD (mg/m²)	Dose Intensity (mg/m²/wk)
NCI/CCSG	24 h CIV q3w	5.5	1.8
St. Jude	3d CIV q3w	1.6	1.6

Note: NCI/CCSG = Children's Cancer Study Group.

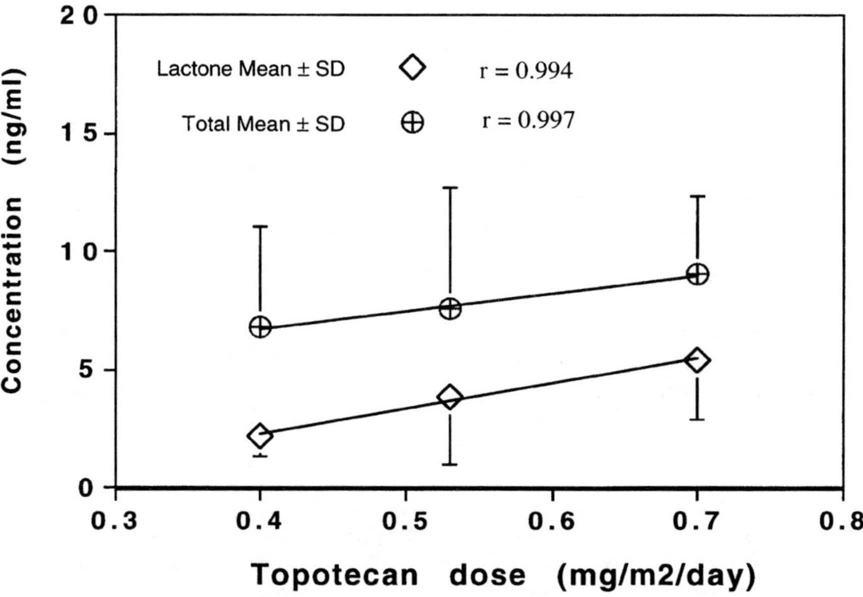

Figure 2 Steady-state concentration of topotecan when given by continuous 21-day infusion.[23]

Steady-state concentrations increased linearly with dose and, as in other studies, lactone accounted for approximately 33% of total drug.

In summary, pharmacokinetic studies done at various institutions are in general agreement concerning the distribution, metabolism, and excretion of topotecan. Blood levels have best fit a two-compartment model in all cases, with beta half-life of 3.0 to 3.5 hours. Pharmacokinetics have been linear with dose as shown in both adults and children, with the drug administered over 30 minutes or 24 hours. For infusion studies, steady-state concentrations have varied with dose but have been determined to range from 2–7 ng/ml at the doses tolerated with acceptable toxicity.

III. CONCLUSIONS AND FUTURE ISSUES

Topotecan is an analog of the plant-derivative camptothecin, a drug which was abandoned in the 1970s due to a perceived poor therapeutic index. Topotecan was synthesized to improve water solubility and to favor formation of the lactone form at physiologic pH.

Clinical studies to date have been carried out with a variety of schedules and doses. The Phase I studies have demonstrated that it is possible safely to administer topotecan as a short (30-minute) bolus infusion every three weeks, by 24-hour infusion every three weeks, and by prolonged infusion from three to twenty-one days. Remarkably, some clinical responses have been seen in heavily pretreated, typical Phase I patients in many of the studies. Pharmacokinetic studies have shown good agreement as to the metabolism and handling of topotecan.

These studies have opened the door to clinical investigation of topotecan, but many unresolved issues remain to be sorted out. Presently, Phase II studies are being conducted to identify the malignant diseases where topotecan will have greatest activities (Tables 5-6). These studies are currently in progress under the auspices of SmithKline and the NCI. Other directions include the use of topotecan in combination with cisplatin, etoposide or taxol; some trials are already in progress using (Table 4). Further studies will investigate the role of newer growth factors (e.g., IL-3 or PIXY-321) to protect against dose-limiting myelosuppression in short administration schedules. High-dose studies in leukemic patients suggest that escalating the dose beyond this toxicity will reveal mucositis as dose-limiting.

Finally, the issue of dose-dependent scheduling remains to be addressed. The Phase I studies clearly demonstrate a dose-dependent toxicity profile, with longer infusions producing dose-limiting myelosuppression at lower doses. Nonetheless, these schedules appear to produce at least equal, if not greater, dose intensity due to duration of infusion. Low-dose infusions may produce less toxicity by yielding blood levels below a threshold for bone marrow suppression or by altering the ratio of the carboxylate to lactone assuming bone marrow toxicity is indeed proportional to the total-drug AUC. Ultimately, will longer infusions produce higher response rates? This question requires further Phase II testing. Promising activity has been seen with prolonged infusion, suggesting dose-dependent activity may be a real issue with this agent. Phase III trials comparing various schedules will be required for determination of the optimal method of topotecan administration. Such comparative trials may also be needed for other inhibitors of topoisomerase-1.

Topotecan is another compound in a new class of anticancer chemotherapy drugs with a novel mechanism of action to have reached the clinic. This drug has been rationally synthesized to overcome problems associated with the parent compound, camptothecin sodium salt, and offers new therapeutic promise, though the challenging issues of schedule and activity remain to be investigated.

REFERENCES

1. **Wall, M. E., Wani, M. C., Cook, C. E., Palmer, K. H., McPhail, A. T., and Sim, G. A.,** Plant antitumor agents: the isolation and structure of camptothecin a novel alkaloidal leukemia and tumor inhibitor from *Camptotheca acuminata. J. Amer. Chem. Soc.*, 88:3888-3890, 1966.

2. **Gottlieb, J. A., Guarino, A. M., Call, J. B., Oliverio, V. T., and Block, J. B.,** Preliminary pharmacological and clinical evaluation of camptothecin sodium (NSC-100880). *Cancer Chemother. Rep.*, 54:461-470, 1970.

3. **Muggia, F. M., Creaven, P. J., Hanson, H. H., Cohen, M. N., and Selawry, O. S.,** Phase I clinical trials of weekly and daily treatment with camptothecin (NSC-100880). Correlation with clinical studies. *Cancer Chemother. Rep.*, 56:515-521, 1972.

4. **Hsiang, Y.-H., Hertzberg, R., Hecht, S., and Liu, L. F.,** Camptothecin induces protein-linked DNA breaks by mammalian DNA topoisomerase-1. *J. Biol. Chem.*, 260:14873-14878, 1985.

5. **Hsiang, Y.-H. and Liu, L. F.,** Identification and mammalian DNA topoisomerase I as an intracellular target of the anticancer drug camptothecin. *Cancer Res.*, 48:1722-1726, 1988.

6. **Jaxel, C., Kohn, K. W., Wani, M. C., Wall, M. E., and Pommier, Y.,** Structure-activity study of the actions of camptothecin derivatives on mammalian DNA topoisomerase-1: evidence for a specific receptor site and a relation to antitumor activity. *Cancer Res.*, 49:1465-1469, 1989.

7. **Hsiang, Y.-H., Liu, L. F., Wall, M. E., Wani, M. C., Nicholas, A. W., Manikumar, G., Kirschenbaum, S., Silber, R., and Potmesil, M.,** DNA topoisomerase I-mediated DNA cleavage and cytotoxicity of camptothecin analogues. *Cancer Res.*, 49:4385-4389, 1989.

8. **Wall, M. E. and Wani, M. C.,** Chemistry and antitumor activity of camptothecins. In Potmesil M. and Kohn K., Eds., *Topoisomerases in Cancer*, Oxford University Press, 1991.

9. **Hertzberg, R. P., Caranfa, M. J., Kingsbury, W. D., Smith, B., Johnson, R. K., and Hecht, S. M.,** The biochemistry of camptothecin-topoisomerase 1 interaction. In *Inhibitors of Topoisomerase 1*. Proc. 2nd Intl. Conf. Topoisomerase in Cancer Chemotherapy. Potmesil, M. and Kohn K., Eds., 103-120, 1990.

10. **Johnson, R. K., Hertzberg, R. P., Eng, W.-K., McCabe, F. L., Kingsbury, W. D., and Hecht, S. M.,** Discovery and design of topoisomerase I inhibitors. *Proc. Am. Soc. Clin. Oncol.*, May 17–19, 1992.

11. **Kingsbury, W. D., Boehm, J. C., Jakas, D. J., Holden, K. G., Hecht, S. M., Gallagher, G., Caranfa, M. J., McCabe, F. L., Faucette, L. F., Johnson, R. K., and Hertzberg, R. P.,** Synthesis of water-soluble (aminoalkyl) camptothecin analogs: inhibition of topoisomerase 1 and antitumor of activity. *J. Med. Chem.*, 34:98-107, 1991.

12. SmithKline Beecham: *Topotecan*, SKF 104864A- Investigator Brochure, March, 1992.

13. **Rowinsky, E., Grochow, L., Hurowitz, L., and Donehower, R.,** Phase I and pharmcologic studies of topotecan, a novel topoisomerase I inhibitor without and with G-CSF. *Seventh NCI-EORTC Symp. New Drugs in Cancer Therapy*, (099), Amsterdam, 1992.

14. **Rowinsky, E., Sartorius, S., Grochow, L., Forastiere, A., Lubejko, B., Hurowitz, L., and Donehower, R.,** Phase I + pharmacology study of topotecan, an inhibitor of topoisomerase 1, with granulocyte colony-stimulating factor (G-CSF): toxicologic differences between concurrent & post-treatment G-CSF administration. *Proc. Am. Soc. Clin. Oncol.*, May 17–19, 1992.

15. **Rowinsky, E. K., Grochow, L. B., Hendricks, C. B., Ettinger, D. S., Forastiere, A. A., Hurowitz, L. A., McGuire, W. P., Sartorius, S. E., Lubejko, B. G., Kaufmann, S. H., and Donehower, R. C.,** Phase I and pharmacologic study of topotecan: a novel topoisomerase 1 inhibitor. *J. Clin.Oncol.*, 10:647-656, 1992.

16. **Saltz, L., Sirott, M., Young, C., Tong, W., Niedzwiecki, D., Tzy-Jyun, Y., Tao, Y., Trochanowski, B., Wright, B., Barbosa, K., Toomasi F, and Kelsen D.,** Phase I clinical and pharmacology study of topotecan given daily for 5 consecutive days to patients with advanced solid tumors, with attempt at dose intensification using recombinant granulocyte colony-stimulating factor. *J. Natl. Cancer. Inst.*, 85: 1499-1506, 1993.

17. **Recondo, G., Abbruzzese, J., Newman, B., Newman, R., Kuhn, J., Von Hoff, D., Garaiz, D., and Raber, M.,** A Phase I trial of topotecan (topo) administered by a 24-hour infusion. *Proc. Am. Assoc. Cancer Res.*, 32:206 (1229), 1991.

18. **Abbruzzese, J., Schmidt, S., Newman, R., and Raber, M.,** Phase I trial of topotecan (topo) administered by a 24-hour infusion. *Seventh NCI-EORTC Symp. New Drugs in Cancer Therapy*, (096), Amsterdam, 1992.

19. **Reid, J. M., Burch, P. A., Benson, L. M., Gilbert, J. A., Richardson, R. L., and Ames, M. M.,** Phase I clinical and pharmacologic evaluation of topotecan administered by a 24-hour continuous infusion. *Proc. Am. Assoc. Cancer Res.*, San Diego, May 1992.

20. **Haas, N. B., Ozols, R. F., and O'Dwyer, P. J.,** Phase I trial of topotecan on a weekly 24-hour infusional schedule. *Seventh NCI-EORTC Symp. New Drugs in Cancer Therapy*, (103), Amsterdam, 1992.

21. **Haas, N. B., LaCreta, F. P., Walczak, J., Hudes, G. R., Brennan, J., Ozols, R. F., and O'Dwyer, P. J.,** Phase I/pharmacokinetic trial of topotecan on a weekly 24-hour infusional schedule. *Proc. Am. Assoc. Cancer Res.*, San Diego, May 1992.

22. **Burris, H., Kuhn, J., Wall, J., Eckardt, J., Rodriguez, G., Johnson, R., Weiss, G., Shaffer, and Von Hoff, D.,** Early clinical trials of topotecan, a new topoisomerase inhibitor. *Seventh NCI-EORTC Symp. New Drugs in Cancer Therapy*, (236), Amsterdam, 1992.

23. **Eckardt, J., Burris, H., Kuhn, J., Smith, S., Rodriguez, G., Weiss, G., Smith, L., Shaffer, D., Johnson, R., and Von Hoff, D.,** Phase I and pharmacokinetic trial of continuous infusion topotecan in patients with refractory solid tumors. *Proc. Am. Soc. Clin. Oncol.*, May 17–19, 1992.

24. **Hochster, H., Speyer, J. S., Oratz, R. O., Meyers, M. M., Wernz, J. C., Chachoua, A., Raphael, B., Sorich, J., Liebes, L., Fry, D., and Blum, R.,** Topotecan 21-day infusion-excellent tolerance of a novel schedule. *Proc. Am. Soc. Clin. Oncol.*, 12:139, 1993.

25. **Hochster, H., Liebes, L., Speyer, J. S., Taubes, B., Oratz, R. O., Wernz, J. C., Chachoua, A., Raphael, B., Vinci, R. Z., Sorich, J., and Blum, R.,** Phase I trial of low-dose, continuous topotecan infusion (7 to 21 days) — an active and well-tolerated regimen. *J. Clin. Oncol.*, March 1994 (in press).

26. **Giovanella, B. C., Wall, M. E., Wani, M. C., Nicholas, A. W., Liu, L. F., Silber, R., and Potmesil, M.,** Highly effective topoisomerase-I targeted chemotherapy of human colon cancer in xenografts. *Science* (Washington, D.C.), 246:1046-1048, 1989.

27. **Kantarjian, H. M., Beran, M., Ellis, A., Zwelling, L., O'Brien, S., Cazenave, L., Koller, C., Rios, M. B., Plunkett, W., and Keating, M. J.,** Phase I Study of Topotecan, a new topoisomerase-1 inhibitor, in patients with refractory or relapsed acute leukemia. *Blood*, 81: 1146-1151, 1993.

28. **Beijnen, J. H., Smith, B. R., Keijer, W. J., van Gijn, R., ten Bokkel Huinink, W. W., Vlasveld, L. T., Rodenhuis, S., and Underberg, W. J.,** High-performance liquid chromatographic analysis of the new antitumor drug SK&F 104864-A in plasma. *J. Pharm. Biomed. Anal.*, 8:789-794, 1990.

29. **Kuhn, J., Burris, H., Irvin, R., Wall, J., Rodriguez, G., Weiss, G., Feilds, S., Hyman, J., Smith, B., Johnson, R., Mann, W., and Von Hoff, D.,** Pharmacokinetics of topotecan following a 30-minute infusion or 3-day continuous infusion. *Seventh NCI-EORTC Symp. New Drugs in Cancer Therapy*, (100), Amsterdam, 1992.

30. **Wall, J. G., Burris, H. A., Von Hoff, D., Rodriquez, G., Kenuper-Hall, R., Shaffer, D., O'Rourke, T., Brown, T., Weiss, G., Clark, G., McVea, S., Brown, R., Johnson, R., Friedman, C., Smith, B., Mann, W., and Kuch, J. A.,** A phase I clinical and pharmacokinetic study of the topoisomerase 1 inhibitor topotecan (SK&F 104864) given as an intravenous bolus every twenty-one days. *Anticancer Drugs*, 3:337-345, 1992

31. **Cole, D., Blaney, S., Balis, F., Reaman, G., Craig, C., Feusner, J., Dinndorf, P., Krailo, M., Ames, M., Hammond, D., and Poplack, D.,** A phase I and pharmacologic study of topotecan in pediatric patients. *Proc. Am. Soc. Clin. Oncol.*, May 17–19, 1992.

Chapter 10

Clinical Trials of Topotecan in Europe

Jaap Verweij, Wim ten Bokkel Huinink, Birthe Lund, André Planting, Jos Beijnen, Maureen de Boer-Dennert, Hilde Rosing, Ineke Koier, and Heine Hansen

CONTENTS

I. INTRODUCTION

Topotecan (SKF 104864-A, NSC 609699) is a semisynthetic analog of camptothecin.[1-3] Camptothecin is known to act by inhibition of topoisomerase I.[4-6] Its development was discontinued because of rather unpredictable side effects. Compared to camptothecin, topotecan has increased hydrophilicity and greatly reduced binding to plasma proteins, expected to result in a decreased and less unpredictable toxicity. Topotecan was highly effective in murine solid tumors and leukemias and in human tumor xenografts.[7] Based on these data, topotecan was selected for clinical trials by the EORTC New Drug Development Committee.

The toxicity of topotecan in animals consisted mainly of myelosuppression and gastrointestinal epithelial cell necrosis. The LD_{10} in mice was 13 mg/m^2/d given for five days. In beagle dogs, this dose was lethal, and a nontoxic dosage was not found. In view of this, the recommended starting dose for Phase I studies was 1/30 of mouse LD_{10}, resulting in a starting dose of 0.5 mg/m^2/d for five consecutive days. For the 24-hour infusion regimen, the starting dose was 2.5 mg/m^2, yielding an equal total dose per course. We performed Phase I studies with topotecan daily times five as short-term infusion (Rotterdam/ Copenhagen), and day 1 24-hour infusion (Amsterdam), in patients with solid tumors with the objectives to:

1. Determine the maximum tolerated dose (MTD) of topotecan in these schedules
2. Determine the qualitative and quantitative toxic effects and to study predictability, duration, intensity, onset, and reversibility of the side effects
3. Recommend the dose for Phase II studies for each schedule
4. Study the pharmacokinetics of topotecan at the different dose levels; and
5. Detect any possible antitumor activity

II. PATIENTS AND METHODS

Eligibility criteria included a histologically confirmed diagnosis of a solid tumor no longer amenable to established forms of treatment; age 18–75 years; WHO performance score 2, life expectancy of 12 weeks; WBC > 4 $\times$ 10^9/l and platelets 100 x 10 ^{9}/l; normal serum bilirubin and – creatinine; no prior history of hemorrhagic cystitis. All patients gave informed consent.

The appropriate dosage of topotecan (SmithKline and Beecham) was diluted in 500 ml of normal saline and administered i.v. by an infusion over 24 hours, repeated every three weeks; or dissolved in 50 ml of normal saline and administered i.v. by infusion pump over 30 minutes, daily for five consecutive days, repeated every three weeks. The starting doses were 2.5 mg/m^2 and 0.5 mg/m^2/d, respectively. Dose escalation was performed in a modified Fibonacci scheme; intrapatient dose escalation was performed in two patients, only in the 24-hour infusion study.

Prior to therapy, a medical history was taken and complete physical examination, hematology screen, and serum chemistries were performed, as were urinalysis, stool guiac test, creatinine clearance, ECG, and chest x-ray. All tests were repeated prior to each subsequent course. Weekly evaluations between courses included history and physical examination, hematology, serum chemistries, urinalysis, and (first week only) stool guiac test. At the highest dose level, hematologic values were evaluated twice a week. All toxicities observed were graded according to WHO criteria. Every second course, tumor parameters were evaluated in patients with measurable lesions; response was defined according to WHO criteria. Patients were taken off study in case of disease progression at evaluation.

The HPLC method used for the analysis of topotecan (SK&F 104864-A) and its lactone ring openend form (SK&F 105992) was developed by Beijnen et al.[8] Whole blood samples were taken before and during the infusion, and at 1, 6, 12, or 18 and 24 hours during the infusion, and at 15, 30, and 60 minutes and 2, 3, 4, 6, 8, 14, 18, and 24 hours afterwards.

III. RESULTS

A. 24-HOUR INFUSION

A total of 26 patients were entered on study. Patient characteristics are given in Table 1. The total number of courses given was 73.

The main toxicities encountered were myelotoxicity (Tables 2 and 3). At the first dose level, already one patient developed a Grade 4 thrombocytopenia. At the following dose levels, mainly at the lower doses, myelotoxicity remained rather unpredictable, although it never became severe. At the two highest dose levels, myelotoxicity was pronounced, while MTD was reached at 10.5 mg/m^2 with both leucocytopenia and thrombocytopenia as dose-limiting factors. The nadir of both leucocytopenia and thrombocytopenia was between day 8 and 15. The duration of severe leuco- and thrombocytopenia was usually short with recovery to Grade 2 within five days. There were no data suggesting cumulative myelotoxicity. Infections during leucocytopenia were not observed.

Mild anemia occurred in 20 patients (77%) and was thought, at least, in part to be related to topotecan administration. Grade 1–3 nausea and vomiting was found not to be dose-dependent and occurred in 27 courses (37%), in 19 courses (26%) being Grade 2 or 3, easily responding to standard anti-emetics in most patients. Alopecia was also not depending on dose and occurred in 20 patients (77%), being total in ten patients (38%). Other incidental side effects were microscopic hematuria (five courses, 7%) and positive stool guiac tests (six courses, 8%). Tumor responses were not observed.

A typical example of the plasma concentration — time curves of topotecan and its lactone-ring openend metabolite are shown in Figure 1. During infusion, the concentrations of both compounds increase and reach maximal levels at the end of infusion. After

Table 1 **Topotecan phase I study: patient characteristics**

	24-h Infusion	D × 5
Total Entered	**26**	**48**
Male/female	14/12	31/17
Age (years)		
Median	53	56
Range	34–67	25–75
PS (WHO)		
Median	1	1
Range	0–2	0–2
Prior Therapy		
Radiotherapy only	1	0
Chemotherapy only	14	24
Radio- and chemotherapy	8	11
None	3	13
Tumor Types		
Colorectal	11	8
Lung (non-small cell)	3	12
Unknown primary	3	3
Soft tissue sarcoma	0	7
Ovary	3	1
Miscellaneous	6	17

Table 2 **Topotecan phase I studies: leukocytopenia**

24 h-Infusion			D × 5		
Dose (mg/m^2)	**Nr of Pts/ Courses**	**WHO Grades 1 2 3 4**	**Dose (mg/m^2/d)**	**Nr of Pts/ Courses**	**WHO Grade 1 2 3 4**
2.50	5/20	1 1 – –	0.50	4/18	1 1 – –
3.75	5/15	2 3 3 –	0.65	6/30	– 21 3 –
5.60	4/11	5 – – –	0.90	11/65	2 11 24 2
8.40	6/13	4 4 3 1	1.00	7/19	1 5 1 1
10.50	5/13	1 1 7 3	1.25	7/41	9 7 9 –
			1.50	12/41	4 5 23 6

cessation of the 24-hour infusion, the concentration of topotecan rapidly declines in a biphasic manner with half-lives: t1/2 (α) 25 min and t1/2 (β) 250 min. Total body clearance (CL_{tot}), calculated as Dose divided by Area Under the plasma concentration time Curve (AUC) from t = 0 to infinity is 0.62 L/min/m^2. The plasma concentrations of the lactone-ring opened metabolite decline in parallel with the parent drug. A linear relationship between the AUC of topotecan and Dose exists in the range 2.5 mg/m^2 – 8.4 mg/m^2. At the higher dose level of 10.5 mg/m^2, the AUCs of topotecan and its metabolite deviate from this linear relationship suggesting a nonlinear pharmacokinetic behavior of the drug when given in these high dosages.

Table 3   **Topotecan phase I studies: thrombocytopenia**

| 24 Hr-Infusion | | | D × 5 | | |
Dose (mg/m²)	Nr of Pts/ Courses	WHO Grades 1 2 3 4	Dose (mg/m²/d)	Nr of Pts/ Courses	WHO Grade 1 2 3 4
2.50	5/20	– – – 1	0.50	4/18	– – 1 –
3.75	5/15	1 4 2 –	0.65	6/30	– – – –
5.60	4/11	– – – –	0.90	11/65	2 11 24 2
8.40	6/13	– 3 2 –	1.00	7/19	1 – 4 –
10.50	5/13	2 1 1 3	1.25	7/41	2 3 2 1
			1.50	12/41	15 4 1 –

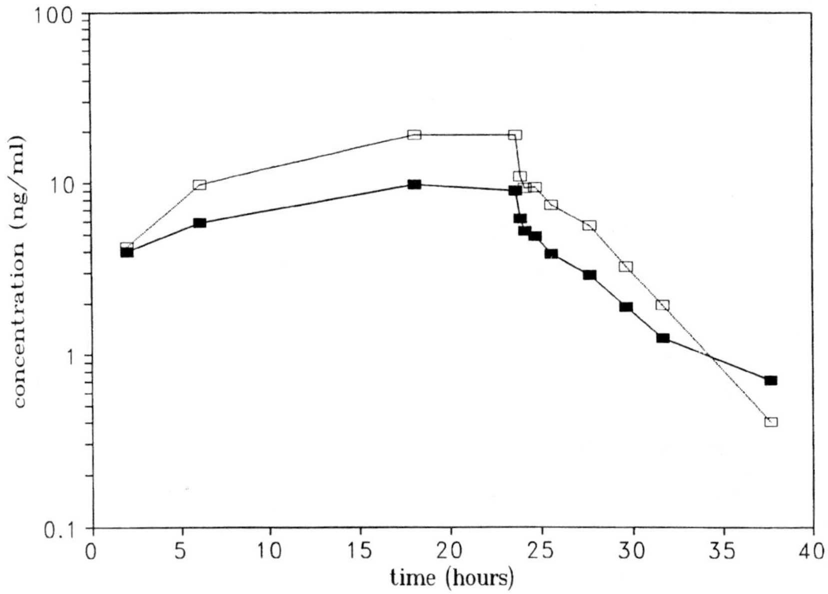

Figure 1   Plasma concentration – time curves of topotecan (■) and its lactone-ring opened form (□). Patient treated with 8.4 mg/m² (total dose: 13.9 mg) of topotecan by continuous infusion over 24 h.

B. DAILY TIMES 5 REGIMEN

A total of 48 patients were entered on study. Patient characteristics are given in Table 1. One patient was not eligible because of poor renal function. The total number of courses evaluated was 214. The median number of courses per patient was four (range 1–24). Two patients could not be evaluated due to non-drug related early death.

The main toxicities encountered were myelotoxicity (Tables 2 and 3). The first patient entered developed a Grade 3 thrombocytopenia, for which reason dose escalation was performed slowly. At the dose of 0.90 mg/m²/d, the leucocytopenias encountered in the first ten courses qualified for maximum tolerated dose. Because of the lack of infectious episodes complicating leucopenia, further experience was obtained at this dose level, and as it was fully uncomplicated, the dose was escalated further (Table 2). At 1.0 and 1.25

mg/m^2/d, severe leucocytopenia was infrequent. At the dose of 1.50 mg/m^2/d, hematologic parameters were taken twice weekly. Granulocytopenia was found to be more marked than leucocytopenia. The nadir of both leucocytopenia and granulocytopenia was between day 8 and 15 with recovery to Grade 2 within five days. Neutropenic fever with lethal infection was observed in one patient at this dose level The dose of 1.50 mg/m^2/d was considered the MTD. Leucocytopenia was difficult to predict at the start of the first course. Previous treatment could not be identified as risk factor. However, the pattern of myelosuppression during the first course in any patient was found to be repetitive in all subsequent courses. Thrombocytopenia (Table 3) was much less frequent and less severe. Anemia occurred frequently but was only incidentally severe. Nausea and vomiting (Grade 1–3) was found to be independent of dose and occurred in 49 courses (23%) in 29 courses (13%) being Grade 2 or 3. Alopecia occurred in nine patients (19%) at all levels, being total in five patients (10%). Other incidental side effects were symptomless hypotension (16%), mild proteinuria (4%), and microscopic hematuria (3%).

Partial responses were seen in three female patients with (pretreated) small cell lung cancer, (pretreated) non-small cell lung cancer, and (non-pretreated) metastatic pancreatic cancer, respectively, lasting 240, 210, and 130 days, respectively. Stable disease was seen in 24 patients.

From 19 patients, complete plasma concentration-time curves were obtained, 15 of which both on day 1 and day 4 or 5. Figure 2 depicts the curves of topotecan and its lactone-ring opened metabolite at the dose of 1.5 mg/m^2, recommended for Phase II studies. Pharmacokinetics were linear and could best be described with an open two-compartment model. The parameters were t1/2alpha 8.1 ± 7.6 min (range 0.3–40.7), t1/2β 132 ± 48 min (range 49–286), $V_{d,ss}$ 72.7 ± 26.9 L/m^2 (range 28.5–123.5), MRT 132 ± 48 min and CL_{tot} 0.57 ± 0.16 L/min/m^2.

IV. CONCLUSION

Topotecan is a semisynthetic derivative of campthotecin, functioning as inhibitor of topoisomerase I.[10] The lactone moiety is essential for this function.[11,12] Cytotoxicity is related to the induced DNA cleavage. Because of this mechanism of action, these drugs are cell cycle-specific, while the readily reversible induced stabilization of the topoisomerase I cleavable complex may result in a schedule dependency. Several studies in tumor models appear to be confirmative in this respect.[13-15] For this reason, the clinical EORTC studies focused on continuous infusion or frequent daily bolus dosing regimen. In animal models, topotecan was superior or equivalent to camptothecin,[11,16] while the major toxicity was reversible myelotoxicity. The recommended starting dose for Phase I studies using a daily times five schedule was 0.5 mg/m^2/d, the starting dose for the Phase I study with the 24-hour infusion was 2.5 mg/m^2. Thus, the total starting dose per course was equal in the two studies. In both Phase I studies, Grade 3 or 4 myelotoxicity was observed at the first dose level, for which reason further dose escalation was performed with relatively small steps. The dose-limiting toxicities of topotecan were leucocytopenia/granulopenia for the daily times five regimen and leucocytopenia plus thrombocytopenia for the 24-hour infusion. The occurrence of these side effects already at the first dose level supports the selection of the conservative starting dose for these studies in view of interspecies differences in animal toxicology.

In the daily times five study, the ten first courses at the dose of 0.9 mg/m^2/d resulted in frequent Grade 3 or 4 leucocytopenia, officially qualifying this dose as MTD. However, because of the lack of infectious episodes complicating this leucocytopenia, the difficult predictability of the occurrence of leucocytopenia, and the known results from a similar Phase I study,[9] the experience at this dose level was further extended. Because

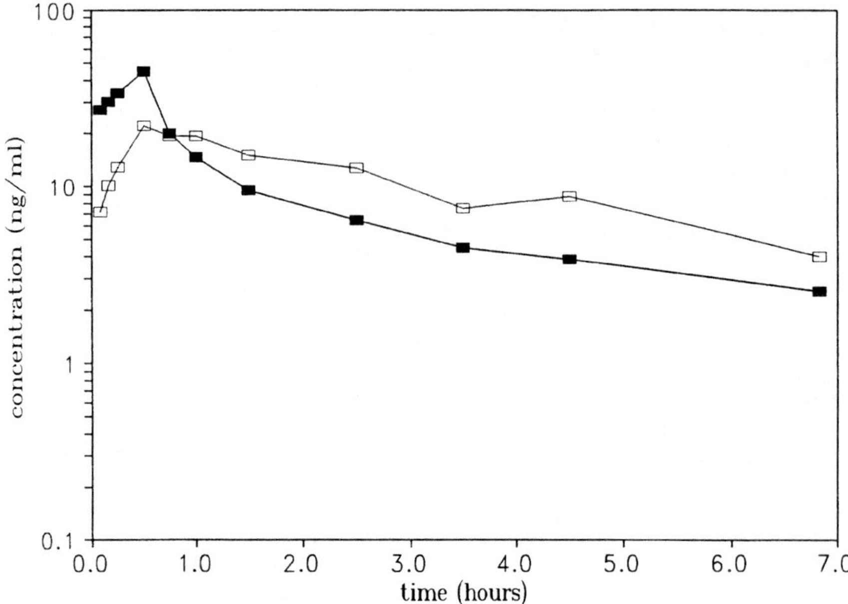

Figure 2   Plasma concentration – time curves of topotecan (■) and its lactone-ring opened form (□). Patient treated with 1.5 mg/m² (total dose: 2.2 mg) of topotecan by 30 min infusion.

finally leucocytopenia in the total 65 courses at this dose level was less pronounced than the initial experience, the dose was escalated further. At the doses of 1.0 mg/m²/d and 1.25 mg/m²/d, Grade 3 or 4 leucocytopenia was less frequent. At the dose of 1.50 mg/m²/d, more than 70% of the courses resulted in Grade 3 or 4 leucocytopenia, and only three courses did not result in leucocytopenia. Besides, 76% of courses resulted in Grade 3 or 4 granulocytopenia, and there were two cases of sepsis, one of which was lethal, during myelosuppression. Thrombocytopenia was less frequent and uncomplicated. The dose of 1.5 mg/m²/d was considered the MTD. In view of the short duration of the nadir and the intrapatient predictability of leucocytopenia during subsequent courses, this dose was also recommended for Phase II studies. Six out of the 13 patients at the dose of 1.5 mg/m²/d were not pretreated with myelosuppressive drugs or extensive radiotherapy, whereas seven had such pretreatment. Nevertheless, leucocytopenia was equally frequent in both groups, for which reason the recommended dose for Phase II studies is similar.

Problems of unpredictability of toxicity at lower doses were also encountered in the 24-hour infusion study. Nevertheless, in this study, the grade of toxicity was more clearly related to dose. In this study, leucocytopenia was also a dose-limiting factor, but it coincided with dose-limiting thrombocytopenia in contrast to the daily times five regimen. The MTD was 10.5 mg/m², at which dose level four out of five patients experienced Grade 3 or 4 leucocytopenia and three out of five patients had Grade 3 or 4 thrombocytopenia. The recommended dose for Phase II studies for this regimen is 8.4 mg/m².

In both studies, anemia was frequent and clearly drug-related. The nonhematological toxicities were generally mild and infrequent. Non-dose-dependent nausea and vomiting (23% in the daily times five study, 37% with the 24-hour infusion) and alopecia (19% and

77%, respectively) were the most frequent. The nausea/vomiting was easily treatable by low-dose standard anti-emetics and did not require 5HT3-antagonist intervention. Although microscopic hematuria and mild proteinuria were incidental findings, there was no evidence for any hemorrhagic cystitis, the second major side effect of sodium camptothecin. Whether this difference is related to the difference in water solubility of these two drugs remains speculative.

The antitumor activity observed in the two similar Phase I studies with the daily times five schedule (seven responses in 77 patients) is encouraging. In addition to the three partial remissions we observed, 24 patients (60% of evaluable patients) had stable disease which is an uncommon experience in Phase I studies.

In view of the fact that all responses were seen with the daily times five regimen which in addition had a slightly more favorable toxicity profile in comparison to the 24-hour infusion schedule, the multiple-day regimen was selected for Phase II studies.

In July 1992, the EORTC Early Clinical Trials Group initiated a Phase II study with topotecan 1.5 mg/m^2/d, day 1–5 once every three weeks in patients with colorectal cancer not pretreated with chemotherapy and in October 1992 a similar study in patients with pretreated small-cell lung cancer. These studies are presently ongoing.

In conclusion, topotecan is an interesting semisynthetic analog of camptothecin, inhibiting topoisomerase I. The antitumor activity seen in Phase I studies using the daily times 5 regimen is noteworthy. Toxicity mainly consists of short-lasting and, most of the time, uncomplicated leucocytopenia. These data support further testing of the drug in Phase II studies.

REFERENCES

1. **Gottlieb, J. A., Guarino, A. M., Call, J. B., Oliverio, V. T., and Block, J. B.,** Preliminary pharmacologic and clinical evaluation of camptothecin sodium (NSC 100880). *Cancer Chemo. Rep.,* 54: 461-470, 1970.

2. **Muggia, F. M., Creaven, P. J., Hansen, H. H., Cohen, M. H., and Selawry, O. S.,** Phase I clinical trial of weekly and daily treatment with camptothecin (NSC 100880): correlation with preclinical studies. *Cancer Chemo. Rep.,* 56: 515-521, 1972.

3. **Creaven, P. J., Allen, L. M., and Muggia, F. M.,** Plasma camptothecin (NSC 100880) levels during a 5-day course of treatment: relation to dose and toxicity. *Cancer Chemo. Rep.,* 56: 573-578, 1972.

4. **Hsiang, Y. H., Hertzberg, R., Hecht, S., and Liu, L. F.,** Camptothecin induces protein-linked DNA breaks via mammalian DNA topoisomerase I. *J. Biol. Chem.,* 260: 14873-14878, 1985.

5. **Hsiang, Y. H. and Liu, L. F.,** Identification of mammalian DNA topoisomerase I as an intracellular target of the anticancer drug camptothecin. *Cancer Res.,* 48: 1722-1726, 1988.

6. **Slichenmyer, W. and Von Hoff, D.,** New natural products in cancer chemotherapy. *J. Clin. Pharmacol.,* 30: 770-788, 1990.

7. **Johnson, R. K., McCabe, F. L., Faucette, L. F., Hertzberg, R. P., Kingberry, W. D., Boehm, J. C., Caranfa, M. J., and Holden, K. G.,** SK&F 104864, a water-soluble analog of camptothecin with broad-spectrum activity in preclinical tumor models. *Proc. AACR,* 30: 623, 1990.

8. **Beijnen, J. H., Smith, B. R., Keijer, W. J., Van Gijn, R., Ten Bokkel Huinink, W. W., Vlasveld, L. Th., Rodenhuis, S., and Underberg, W. J. M.,** High-performance liquid chromatographic analysis of the new antitumor drug SK&F 104864-A (NSC 609699) in plasma. *J. Pharm. Biomed. Anal.,* 8: 789-794, 1990.

9. **Rowinsky, E. K., Grochow, L. B., Hendriks, C. B., Ettinger, D. S., Forastiere, A. A., Horowitz, L. A., McGuire, W. P., Sartorius, S. E., Lubejko, B. G., Kaufmann, S. H., and Donehower, R. C.,** Phase I and pharmacologic study of topotecan: a novel topoisomerase I inhibitor. *J. Clin. Oncol.,* 10: 647-656, 1992.

10. **Hertzberg, R. P., Caranfa, M. J., and Hecht, S. M.,** On the mechanism of topoisomerase I inhibition by camptothecin: evidence for binding to an enzyme-DNA complex. *Biochemistry,* 28: 4629-4638, 1989.

11. **Hertzberg, R. P., Caranfa, M. J., Holden, K. G., Jakas, D. R., Gallagher, G., Mattern, M. R., Mong, S. M., Bartus, J. O., Johnson, R. K., and Kingsbury, W. D.,** Modification of the hydroxy lactone ring of camptothecin: inhibition of mammalian topoisomerase I and biological activity. *J. Med. Chem.,* 32: 715-720, 1989.

12. **Wall, M. E. and Wani, M. C.,** Antineoplastic agents from plants. *Ann. Rev. Pharmacol. Toxicol.,* 17: 117-132, 1977.

13. Data on file at SmithKline Beecham.

14. **Burns, H., Kuhn, J., Johnson, R., and Von Hoff, D.,** SKF 104864: preclinical studies of a new topoisomerase I inhibitor. *Proc. AACR,* 31: 431, 1990.

15. **Houghton, P. J., Cheshire, P. J., Myers, L., and Houghton, J. A.,** Evaluation of 9-dimethylaminomethyl-10-hydroxy camptothecin (topotecan) against xenografts derived from adult and childhood tumors. *Ann. Oncol.,* 3 (suppl 1): 84, 1992.

16. **Johnson, R. K., Hertzberg, R. P., Kingsburry, W. D., Boehm, J. C., Caranfa, M. J., Faucette, L. F., McCabe, F. L., and Holden, K. G.,** Preclinical profile of SKF 104864, a water-soluble analog of camptothecin. *Proc. 6th NCI-EORTC Symp. New Drug in Cancer Therapy,* abstr. 301, 1989.

Chapter 11

Camptothecins: Dose-Limiting Toxicities and Their Management

Howard A. Burris, III, Suzanne M. Fields, John G. Kuhn, and Daniel D. Von Hoff

CONTENTS

I. INTRODUCTION

Camptothecin is a product derived from the stem wood of the Chinese tree *Camptotheca acuminata* that was originally isolated during the National Cancer Institute's natural products screening program in the early 1950s.[1] Because camptothecin demonstrated significant antitumor activity against murine leukemia and sarcoma cell lines, Phase I clinical trials were initiated with the sodium salt of the parent compound in the early 1970s.[2-3] The sodium salt of camptothecin was used in order to increase the solubility of the compound and facilitate intravenous drug administration. Unfortunately, these trials were discontinued prematurely due to unpredictable myelosuppression, gastrointestinal toxicities, and severe hemorrhagic cystitis, despite antitumor responses in patients with gastric and colon cancer. In fact, at the American Association of Cancer Research Meeting in Chicago in 1971, camptothecin was referred to as "a drug of protean and unpredictable toxicity that has no clinical value in the management of gastrointestinal cancer".

Although the clinical development of camptothecin waned, interest in determining the precise mechanism of action continued in the laboratories of Susan Horwitz and David Kessel.[4,5] Camptothecin and its analogs possess a unique mechanism of antitumor action, inhibition of topoisomerase I (see Chapter 1). Based on their mechanism of action, these agents are classified as S-phase specific antineoplastic agents.

The determination of this unique mechanism of action triggered a renewed interest in the development of camptothecin derivatives. As a result, two new compounds, topotecan and irinotecan (CPT-11), were synthesized from the parent compound in an attempt to reduce the toxicities of camptothecin while maintaining or improving the antitumor activity. The structures of the parent compound and the two derivatives are depicted in

Figure 1. Both topotecan and irinotecan have increased water solubility at an acidic pH in order to prevent the development of hemorrhagic cystitis. In an acidic environment, such as the urine, camptothecin sodium is converted to an insoluble closed lactone-ring derivative, which could lead to hemorrhagic cystitis. The new compounds also have decreased protein binding compared to camptothecin, which theoretically could result in more predictable myelosuppression as there is less drug available for protein displacement.[6,7] The remainder of this chapter will focus on the toxicity differences between the compounds, the relationship between the toxicities and the pharmacology and schedule of administration of the drug, and the different supportive care strategies that are needed during treatment.

II. HEMATOLOGIC TOXICITIES OF TROPOTECAN

Topotecan has been extensively tested in Phase I clinical trials in a variety of intravenous schedules including single bolus doses, multiple consecutive daily doses, and continuous infusions of 24, 72, and 120 hours duration. Table 1 summarizes the studies that have been reported to date.[8-24] The dose-limiting toxicity for all of the trials has been myelosuppression, specifically neutropenia and thrombocytopenia. With the shorter infusion schedules, a noncumulative neutropenia has predominated as the dose-limiting effect. The neutropenia is generally short-lived (3–5 days' duration) and resolves spontaneously without growth factor support. However, when the infusion is prolonged to 72 or 120 hours, thrombocytopenia emerges as the dose-limiting toxicity in combination with neutropenia.

Because neutropenia is dose-limiting, Rowinsky and colleagues investigated the combination of topotecan and granulocyte-colony stimulating factor (G-CSF) in an attempt to escalate the maximally tolerated dose.[14] As illustrated in Table 2, the combination of topotecan and G-CSF actually potentiated the neutropenia and thrombocytopenia associated with topotecan when the drug was administered as a daily bolus dose for five days. Therefore, it appears that the combination of G-CSF and topotecan administered as a daily dose for five consecutive days is limited by the development of thrombocytopenia. More recently, Janik et al. explored the combination of topotecan and granuylocyte-macrophage-colony stimulating factor (GM-CSF) administered in two different dosing schedules.[25] Patients with renal cell cancer or melanoma receiving topotecan 1.5 mg/m^2 daily for five days were randomized to receive GM-CSF 250 mcg/m^2 daily for seven days post-topotecan or GM-CSF 250 mcg/m^2 twice daily for five days before chemotherapy plus GM-CSF 250 mcg/m^2 daily for seven days post-topotecan. Seventy-seven percent (10/13) of the patients receiving post-treatment GM-CSF experienced Grade 4 neutropenia, while only 27% (4/11) of the patients receiving GM-CSF pre- and post-chemotherapy developed the same degree of neutropenia. However, no differences were noted in the nadir platelet counts between the two groups. By changing the administration schedule of topotecan and G-CSF or GM-CSF, it may be possible to escalate the dose of topotecan. However, the development of thrombocytopenia may still be a problem with the use of lineage-specific stimulating factors. The use of alternative multi-lineage hematopoietic stimulating factors, such as PIXY (a fusion of granulocyte-macrophage-colony stimulating factor and interleukin-3), may also allow dose intensity in the absence of hematologic toxicities.

In addition to the neutropenia and thrombocytopenia, approximately 20% of patients experienced mild anemia with all of the treatment schedules tested with topotecan. The etiology of the anemia remains unknown.

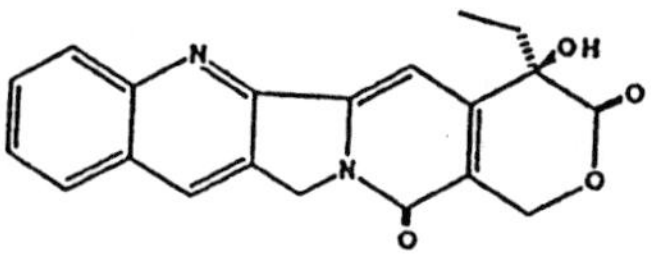

Camptothecin

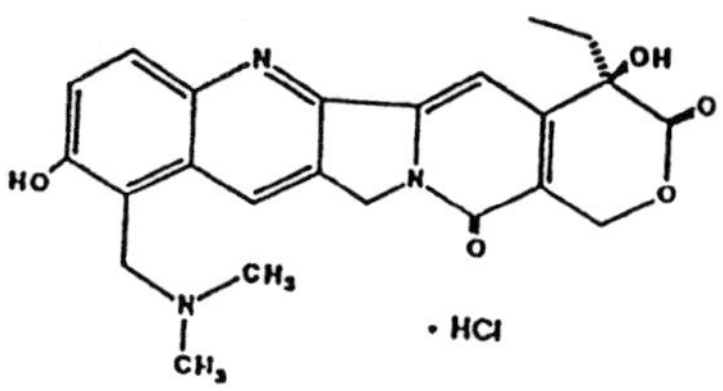

Topotecan

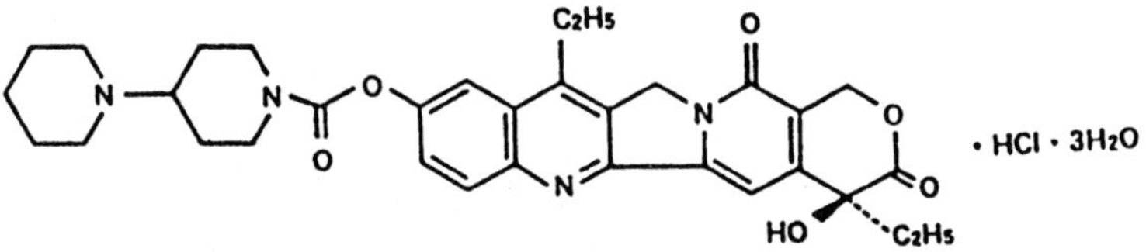

Irinotecan

Figure 1 Chemical structures of camptothecin, topotecan, and irinotecan.

III. PHARMACOLOGY OF TOPOTECAN

Pharmacokinetic studies with topotecan have suggested a correlation between the clinical pharmacology and hematologic toxicities of the drug. In a basic environment, topotecan is rapidly hydrolyzed from the closed lactone form of the molecule to the open carboxylate form (Figure 2). This hydrolysis reaction is important because the closed lactone form of the drug is the only form demonstrating antineoplastic activity in preclinical systems. Following intravenous administration, both the closed lactone form of the drug and the open carboxylate form exhibit biexponential elimination curves with a half-life of approximately 3.4 hours.[8,10] Renal excretion is the primary route of elimination, as 40% of the drug is recovered in the urine during the first 24 hours. Both peak plasma concentration and area under the curve for topotecan have been correlated with the development of neutropenia. Pharmacodynamic studies have also suggested a correlation between the dose of topotecan administered and the percent decrease in a patient's absolute neutrophil count. This relationship is best described by a maximum effect [E_{max}] model.[8,10]

IV. NONHEMATOLOGIC TOXICITIES OF TOPOTECAN

Topotecan administration is also associated with a variety of nonhematologic toxicities that are all relatively mild and do not require special supportive care.[8-24] Gastrointestinal toxicities in the form of nausea (Grades 1 and 2), vomiting (Grade 1), and diarrhea (Grades 1 and 2) have been reported in 20–30% of the patients in the Phase I trials. All of these toxicities are easily controlled with symptomatic therapy, such as standard oral antiemetics and antidiarrheals. Other toxicities which occur in a small percentage of patients include low grade fevers (15%), rash (14%), and fatigue (10%). Alopecia, however, occurs in greater than 80% of patients treated with topotecan. Most importantly, no patients experienced gastrointestinal bleeding or hemorrhagic cystitis with topotecan therapy.

Table 1 **Phase I trials with topotecan**

Schedule	MDT mg/m²/d	Total Dose mg/m²	Dose-Limiting Toxicity	Reference
30 min bolus Q21d	22.5	22.5	Neutropenia	8
30 min bolus Q21d	22.5	22.5	Neutropenia	9
30 min daily × 5 Q21d	2.5	12.5	Neutropenia	10
30 min daily × 5 Q21d	1.5	7.5	Neutropenia	11
30 min daily × 5 Q28d	1.75	8.75	Neutropenia	12
30 min daily × 5 Q21d[†]	1.5	7.5	Thrombocytopenia	13
30 min daily × 5 Q21d[†]	2.5	12.5	Thrombocytopenia Neutropenia	14
24 hour CI weekly	2.0	6.0	Neutropenia	15
24 hour CI Q21d	8.4	8.4	Neutropenia Thrombocytopenia	16
24 hour CI Q21d	10.0	10.0	Neutropenia Thrombocytopenia	17
24 hour CI Q21d[†]	15.0	15.0	Thrombocytopenia	17
24 hour CI Q21d[*]	7.5	7.5	Neutropenia Thrombocytopenia	18
72 hour CI[*]	1.0	3.0	Neutropenia	19
72 hour CI weekly	2.0	6.0	Myelosuppression	20
72 hour CI Q14d	2.6	7.8	Myelosuppression	20
72 hour CI Q21d	1.6	4.8	Neutropenia Thrombocytopenia	21
120 hour CI Q21d	0.68	3.4	Neutropenia Thrombocytopenia	21
120 hour CI Q21–28d	2.0	10.0	Mucositis	22
21 day CI Q28d	0.53	11.13	Neutropenia Thrombocytopenia	23
24 hour CI Q28d IP	4.0	4.0	Neutropenia	24

Note: MTD = Maximally Tolerated Dose; † = with granulocyte-colony stimulating factor: * = pediatric patients; IP = intraperitoneal.

Table 2 **Phase I trial of topotecan administered daily × five days with or without granulocyte-colony stimulating factor (G-CSF)**

	With G-CSF	Without G-CSF
Grade IV neutropenia	78%	37%
Grade IV thrombocytopenia	57%	0%
Median absolute neutrophil count nadir	168	681
Median platelet nadir	64K	147K

From Reference 14.

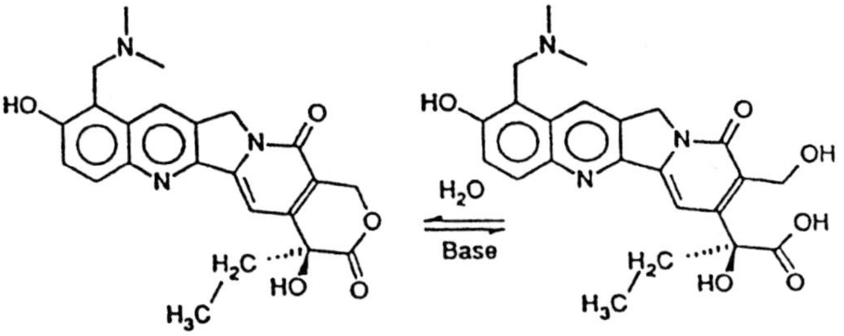

Figure 2 Hydrolysis reaction of topotecan from the closed lactone form (active) to the open carboxylate form (inactive) of the molecule.

V. IRINOTECAN (CPT-11)

The majority of the early clinical development of irinotecan was conducted in Japan. The various Phase I trials reported in the literature are summarized in Table 3. As demonstrated in the table, the dose-limiting toxicities have varied based on the dosing schedule used in the trial. The dose-limiting toxicities have consisted of myelosuppression, primarily neutropenia, and gastrointestinal toxicities, specifically diarrhea. The myelosuppression appears to correlate with the frequency of drug administration as the daily dosing schedules produced more neutropenia and thrombocytopenia. On the other hand, the intermittent schedules which utilize higher single doses of irinotecan have been associated with the development of gastrointestinal toxicities, such as diarrhea. The duration of infusion (30 minutes versus 90 minutes) may also contribute to the toxicities as the shorter infusions have produced more neutropenia than the longer infusions. Furthermore, it may be necessary to include built-in rest periods in the dosing schedules. The schedule tested in San Antonio (weekly $\times$ 4 q six weeks) had a two-week rest period built into the regimen which may contribute to the ability to increase the weekly dose of irinotecan to 180 mg/ m^2 in some patients

VI. PHARMACOLOGY OF IRINOTECAN

As with topotecan, the pharmacology of irinotecan is important in the development of drug toxicities. Irinotecan is actually a pro-drug that is rapidly hydrolyzed by carboxylesterase enzymes to its active metabolite, SN-38, following intravenous administration.[26,27,34] SN-38 has been shown to be at least 100-fold more potent than irinotecan in causing DNA strand breaks.[35] Both irinotecan and SN-38 exist in the open and closed lactone-ring forms, but only the closed lactone-ring forms are active. Therefore, it is important to measure the open and closed lactone-ring forms of both irinotecan and SN-38 in patients' serum following drug administration. Irinotecan elimination exhibits a triexponential pattern with an elimination half-life of approximately 5–7 hours. It is primarily excreted in the feces, as only 25% of the drug is recoverable in the urine following administration. In contrast, the elimination half-life of SN-38 is longer (approximately 11–18 hours), and virtually all of the metabolite is excreted in the bile and feces. Irinotecan also undergoes extensive enterohepatic circulation resulting in second SN-38 peaks following drug administration, which may contribute to the development of diarrhea as the area under the curve (AUC) for SN-38 has been shown to correlate with diarrhea.[36,37] The AUC for irinotecan, on the other hand, has been shown to correlate with the development of neutropenia.

Table 3 **Phase I studies with irinotecan**

Schedule	Infusion Duration	MTD mg/m²/d	Dose Intensity* mg/m²	Dose-Limiting Toxicity	Ref.
Single q 21 d	90 min	240	240	Neutropenia Diarrhea	25
Weekly × 4 q 42 d	90 min	280	360	Diarrhea	26
Weekly	30 min	145	435	Neutropenia	27
QD × 3 q 21 d	30 min	115	345	Neutropenia	28
Single q 21 d	30 min	750	750	Not yet defined	29
CI q 21 d	120 h	40	200	Diarrhea	30
Weekly	90 min	150	450	Leukopenia Diarrhea	31
Single q 28 d	60 min	250	188	Neutropenia	32

Note: MTD = Maximally Tolerated Dose; CI = Continuous Infusion

*Dose administered in a 21-day period in mg/m².

VII. GASTROINTESTINAL TOXICITIES OF IRINOTECAN

The administration of irinotecan has produced a variety of gastrointestinal toxicities including nausea, vomiting, diarrhea, and anorexia. The nausea and vomiting are generally moderate (26% and 15% experience Grade 3 and 4, respectively, based on WHO criteria) and are easily controlled. Irinotecan-induced diarrhea, however, ranges from moderate to severe, with approximately 20% of patients experiencing Grade 3 or 4 diarrhea (WHO criteria). Unfortunately, the development of diarrhea has not been predictable based on any specific patient characteristics. The etiology of the diarrhea is unknown, but it appears to be a parasympathetic reaction. Research conducted at The University of Texas Health Science Center in San Antonio suggests that the development of diarrhea may correlate with the amount of carboxylesterase activity in the intestinal mucosa, liver, and plasma of patients receiving irinotecan. In the data collected to date, patients with high carboxylesterase levels have experienced more diarrhea than other patients. This may be due to increased production of SN-38 from irinotecan in these patients, but this data is still preliminary. Another factor that may contribute to the development of diarrhea with irinotecan is that the drug is formulated in sorbitol, a known laxative. Whether the amount of sorbitol administered with a single intravenous dose or irinotecan is clinically significant remains to be determined. Approximately one-fourth of patients receiving irinotecan will also experience Grade 3 and 4 anorexia.

A broad range of supportive care modalities have been used in the management of irinotecan-induced toxicities. Although the nausea and vomiting is mild to moderate, the use of prophylactic antiemetic premedication is frequently necessary at irinotecan doses 100 mg/m². The administration of a single dose of a serotonin antagonist plus or minus the concomitant administration of a single dose of steroids is quite effective in controlling the nausea and vomiting. Numerous agents including loperamide, diphenhydramine, diphenoxylate, scopolamine, atropine, and somatostatin have been used for the symptomatic treatment of irinotecan-induced diarrhea with various degrees of success. Typically, the diarrhea remains severe for 5 to 7 days before resolution, but prompt initiation of aggressive antidiarrheal therapy at the first sign of loose stools or abdominal cramping may help obviate the severity of the diarrhea. The administration of loperamide at the first sign of diarrhea and repeated as often as every two hours until symptoms are controlled currently appears to be the most effective regimen for the managment of drug-induced diarrhea.

VIII. HEMATOLOGIC TOXICITIES OF IRINOTECAN

Various irinotecan treatment regimens have also been associated with the development of significant neutropenia, thrombocytopenia, and anemia. Approximately 40% of patients in the clinical trials developed Grade 3 and 4 neutropenia. Furthermore, neutropenia was the dose-limiting toxicity in several of the Phase I trials. Because of the nonhematologic toxicities reported with irinotecan dose escalation with growth factor support has not been pursued in the trials reported to date. Severe thrombocytopenia (Grades 3 and 4) is reported in less than 10% of the patients treated with irinotecan, while approximately 20% of patients experience a significant degree of anemia with treatment.

IX. CONCLUSION

Based on their unique mechanism of action, the topoisomerase I inhibitors may be an extremely useful addition to the chemotherapeutic armamentarium. The sodium salt of the parent compound in this series, camptothecin, was associated with severe unpredictable side effects. However, the water-soluble derivatives of camptothecin, specifically topotecan and irinotecan, have been tolerated much better in early clinical trials. Topotecan dosing has been associated with minimal nonhematologic toxicities but has been limited by the development of neutropenia and thrombocytopenia. Clinical trials investigating the use of colony-stimulating factors with topotecan are currently underway in an attempt to eliminate these toxicities. A Phase I trial of oral topotecan is also being conducted in an attempt to take advantage of the pharmacologic properties of the drug and maximize tumor exposure to the active lactone derivative. With irinotecan, the dose-limiting toxicities have varied based on the schedule used for drug administration. However, the primary toxicity limiting drug administration is the unpredictable development of diarrhea. A great deal of research is currently being conducted regarding the etiology of this diarrhea, and numerous supportive care regimens are being investigated in an attempt to ameliorate this toxicity. Phase II trials exploring the specific antitumor activity of these compounds as single agents as well as in combination with other antineoplastic agents are also well underway.

REFERENCES

1. **Wall, M. E., Wani, M. C., Cook, C. E., et al.,** Plant anti-tumor agents. 1. The isolation and structure of camptothecin, a novel alkaloidal leukemia and tumor inhibitor from *Camptotheca acuminata.*, *J. Am. Chem. Soc.*, 88:3888-3890, 1966.
2. **Muggia, F. M., Creven, P. J., Hansen, H. H., et al.,** Phase I clinical trial of weekly an daily treatment with camptothecin (NSC 100880): correlation with preclinical studies. *Cancer Chemother. Rep.*, 56:515-5221, 1972.
3. **Gottlieb, J. A., Guarino, A. M., Call, J. B., et al.,** Preliminary pharmacologic and clinical evaluation of camptothecin sodium (NSC 100880). *Cancer Chemother. Rep.*, 54:461-470, 1970.
4. **Horwitz, S. B. and Horwitz, M. S.,** Effects of camptothecin on the breakage and repair of DNA during the cell cycle. *Cancer Res.*, 33:2834-2836, 1973.
5. **Spataro, A. and Kessel, D.,** The effects of camptothecin on mammalian DNA. *Biochim. Biophys. Acta.*, 331:194-201, 1973.
6. **Hertzberg, R. P., Caranfa, M. J., Holden, K. G., et al.,** Modification of the hydroxy lactone ring of camptothecin: inhibition of mammalian topoisomerase I and biological activity. *J. Med. Chem.*, 32:715-720, 1989.

7. **Kunimoto, T., Nitta, K., Tanaka, T., et al.,** Antitumor activity of 7-ethyl-10[4-(1-piperidino)-1-peperidino] carbonyloxy-camptothecin, a novel water-soluble derivative of camptothecin against murine tumors, *Cancer Res.,* 47:5944-5947, 1987.

8. **Wall, J. G., Burris, H. A., III, H. A., Von Hoff, D. D., et al.,** A phase I clinical and pharmacokinetic study of the topoisomerase I inhibitor topotecan (SK&F 104864) given as an intravenous bolus every 21 days. *Anti-Cancer Drugs,* 3:337-345, 1992.

9. **Hasegawa, K., Nishimura, R., Fukuoka, M., et al.,** Phase I and pharmacologic evaluation of topotecan on a 30-minute infusion. *Proc. Am. Assoc. Cancer Res.,* 34:421, 1993 (abstract).

10. **Rowinsky, E. K., Grochow, L. B., Hendricks, C. B., et al.,** Phase I and pharmacologic study of topotecan: a novel topoisomerase I inhibitor. *J. Clin. Oncol.,* 10:647-565, 1992.

11. **Verweij, J., Lund, B., Beynen, J., et al.,** Clinical studies with topotecan: the EORTC experience. *Ann. Oncol.,* 3(Suppl 1):118, 1992 (abstract).

12. **Saltz, L., Sirott, M., Young, C., et al.,** Phase I and clinical pharmacologic study of intravenous topotecan alone and with granulocyte-colony stimulating factor (G-CSF). *Ann. Oncol.,* 3(Suppl 1):84, 1992 (abstract).

13. **Murphy, B., Saltz, L., Sirott, M., et al.,** Granulocyte-colony stimulating factor (G-CSF) does not increase the maximum tolerated dose (MTD) in a phase I study of topotecan (T). *Proc. Am. Soc. Clin. Oncol.,* 11:139, 1992 (abstract).

14. **Rowinsky, E., Sartorius, S., Grochow, L., et al.,** Phase I & pharmacologic study of topotecan, an inhibitor of topoisomerase I, with granulocyte-colony stimulating factor (G-CSF): toxicologic differences between concurrent & post-treatment G-CSF administration. *Proc. Am. Soc. Clin. Oncol.,* 11:116, 1992 (abstract.

15. **Haas, N. B., Hudes, G. R., Walczak, I., et al.,** Phase I trial of topotecan on a weekly 24-hour infusional schedule. *Ann. Oncol.,* 3(Suppl 1): 84, 1992 (abstract).

16. **ten Bokkel Huinink, W. W., Rodenhuis, S., Beijnen, J., et al.,** Phase I study of the topoisomerase I inhibitor topotecan (SK&F104864-A). *Proc. Am. Soc. Clin. Oncol.,* 11:110, 1992 (abstract).

17. **Abbruzzese, J. L., Madden, T., Schmidt, S., et al.,** Phase I trial of topotecan (TT) administered by 24-hour infusion without and with G-CSF. *Proc. Am. Assoc. Cancer Res.,* 34:329, 1993 (abstract).

18. **Blaney, S. M., Balis, F. M., Cole, D. E., et al.,** Pediatric phase I trial and pharmacokinetic study of topotecan administered as a 24-hour continuous infusion. *Cancer Res.,* 53:1032-1036, 1993.

19. **Pratt, C., Stewart, C., Santana, V., et al.,** Phase I study of topotecan for pediatric patients with drug-resistant solid tumors. *Proc. Am. Soc. Clin. Oncol.,* 12:410, 1993 (abstract).

20. **Sabiers, J. H., Berger, N. A., Berger, S. J., et al.,** Phase I trial of topotecan administered as a 72-hour infusion. *Proc. Am. Assoc. Cancer Res.,* 34:426, 1993 (abstract).

21. **Burris, H., Kuhn, J., Wall, J., et. al.,** Early clinical trials of topotecan, a new topoisomerase I inhibitor. *Ann. Oncol.,* 3(Suppl 1):118, 1992 (abstract).

22. **Kantarjian, H. M., Beran, M., Ellis, A., et al.,** Phase I study of topotecan, a new topoisomerase I inhibitor, in patients with refractory or relapsed acute leukemia. *Blood,* 81:1146-1151, 1993.

23. **Hochster, H., Speyer, J., Oratz, R., et. al.,** Topotecan 21-day continuous infusion-excellent tolerance of a novel schedule. *Proc. Am. Soc. Clin. Oncol.,* 12:139, 1993 (abstract).

24. **Plaxe, S., Christen, R., O'Quigley, J., et al.,** Phase I trial of intraperitoneal topotecan. *Proc. Am. Soc. Clin. Oncol.,* 12:140, 1993 (abstract).

25. **Janik, J., Miller, L., Smith, II, J., et al.,** Prechemotherapy granulocyte-macrophage-colony stimulating factor (GM-CSF) prevents topotecan-induced neutropenia. *Proc. Am. Soc. Clin. Oncol.,* 12:437, 1993 (abstract).

26. **Rowinsky, E., Grochow, L., Ettinger, D., et al.,** Phase I and pharmacologic study of CPT-11, a semisynthetic topoisomerase I-targeting agent, on a single dose schedule. *Proc. Am. Soc. Clin. Oncol.,* 11:115, 1992 (abstract).

27. **Rothenberg, M. L., Kuhn, J. G., Burris, H. A., et al.,** Phase I and pharmacokinetic trial of weekly CPT-11. *J. Clin. Oncol.,* 11:2194-2204, 1993.

28. **Extra, J. M., De Forni, M., Culine, S., et al.,** Phase I of CPT-11, a camptothecin analog, administered as a weekly infusion. *Ann. Oncol.,* 3(Suppl 1):83, 1992 (abstract).

29. **Clavel, M., Mathieu-Boue, A., Dumortier, A., et al.,** Phase I of CPT-11 administered as a daily infusion for 3 consecutive days. *Proc. Am. Assoc., Cancer Res.,* 33:262, 1992 (abstract).

30. **Abigerges, D., Armand, J. P., Chabot, G. G., et al.,** High-dose intensity of CPT-11 administered as a single dose every 3 weeks: the Institut Gustave Roussy experience. *Proc. Am. Soc. Clin. Oncol.,* 12:133, 1993 (abstract).

31. **Ohe, Y., Sasaki, Y., Shinkai, T., et al.,** Phase I study and pharmacokinetics of CPT-11 with 5-day continuous infusion. *J. Natl. Cancer Inst.,* 84:972-974, 1992.

32. **Negoro, S., Fukuoka, M., Masuda, N., et al.,** Phase I study of weekly intravenous infusions of CPT-11, a nedw derivative of camptothecin, in the treatment of advanced non-small cell lung cancer. *J. Natl. Cancer Inst.,* 83:1164-1168, 1991.

33. **Taguchi, T., Wakui, A., Hasegawa, K., et al.,** Phase I clinical study of CPT-11. *Jpn. J. Cancer Chemother.,* 17:115-120, 1990.

34. **Kanzawa, F., Kondoh, H., Kwon, S., et al.,** Role of carboxylesterase on metabolism of camptothecin analog (CPT-11) in non-small cell lung cancer cell line PC-7 cells. *Proc. Am. Assoc. Cancer Res.,* 33:427, 1992 (abstract).

35. **Kawato, Y., Aonuma, M., Hirota, Y., et al.,** Intracellular roles of SN-38, a metabolite of the camptothcin derivative CPT-11, in the antitumor effect of CPT-11. *Cancer Res.,* 51:4187-4191, 1991.

36. **Sasaki, Y., Morita, M., Miya, T., et al.,** Pharmacokinetics (PK) and pharmacodynamic (PD) analysis of CPT-11 and its active metabolite SN-38. *Proc. Am. Soc. Clin. Oncol.,* 11:111, 1992 (abstract).

37. **Kudoh, S., Fukuoka, M., Masuda, N., et al.,** Relationship between CPT-11 pharmacokinetics and diarrhea in the combination chemotherapy of irinotecan (CPT-11) and cisplatin (CDDP). *Proc. Am. Soc. Clin. Oncol.,* 12:141, 1993 (abstract).

Cellular Determinants of Sensitivity and Resistance to Camptothecins

Yves Pommier, Akihiko Tanizawa, Kosuke Okada, and Toshiwo Andoh

CONTENTS

I. INTRODUCTION

A. IMPORTANCE OF TOPOISOMERASE I FOR CANCER CHEMOTHERAPY

DNA topoisomerase I (topo I) is encoded by a single-copy gene located on chromosome 20q12-13.2.[1,2] It is highly expressed in a variety of tumors including chronic lymphocytic leukemia and several types of lymphoma, primary human colon adenocarcinoma,[3] and ovarian tumors.[4] By contrast to topo II, whose expression is tightly linked to cell proliferation, increasing sharply during S-phase before dropping to low level in G1-phase, topo I activity increases only two-fold during the S-phase of the cell cycle[5,6] and is present in nondividing cells.[5-8] This point may be of considerable interest with respect to chemotherapy since a large fraction of tumor cells divide very slowly and, therefore, could be targeted with topo I inhibitors.

Topo I activity is regulated by post-translational modifications. Dephosphorylation abolishes catalytic activity and camptothecin sensitivity,[9-15] while phosphorylation by protein kinase C stimulates activity[14,16] and enhances the formation of topo I-mediated DNA single-strand breaks.[14] This may be why treatment of cells with tumor necrosis factor,[17] hormones, growth factors,[18,19] as well as leukotriene D_4[20] and phorbol esters[14] (Kerrigan and Pommier, unpublished results) rapidly stimulate topo I catalytic activity and camptothecin-induced DNA breaks. By contrast, tyrosine phosphorylation by P60[src] has been shown to inactivate purified topoisomerases *in vitro*.[11] Similarly, poly(ADP-ribosyl)ation of topo I inhibits catalytic activity,[21-28] and pretreatment of cells with the poly(ADPribose) inhibitor, 3-aminobenzamide, increases camptothecin-induced DNA breaks.[29] Other, post-transcriptional modifications, such as interactions with acidic phospholipids[30] and heparin[31] may also down-regulate catalytic activity.

There is good evidence that topo I is the major cellular target of camptothecin: (1) the potency of camptothecin derivatives against purified topo I is correlated with their antitumor activity;[32,33] (2) camptothecin-induced DNA breaks produced in cells exhibit the characteristics of topo I-linked DNA breaks;[29,34,35] (3) camptothecin-resistant cells fail to produce topo I-linked DNA breaks and contain either camptothecin-resistant topo I or reduced topo I levels (see next section); (4) yeast mutants lacking the endogenous topo I gene are camptothecin-resistant and can be made drug-sensitive by transfecting the human topo I gene;[36-38] (5) cells transfected with the human topo I gene are hypersensitive to camptothecin;[39] and (6) site-directed mutagenesis of topo I similar to one of the mutations (at Gly-533) observed in camptothecin-resistant CPT-K5 cells yields a camptothecin-resistant enzyme (Andoh et al., manuscript in preparation).

B. CAMPTOTHECIN DERIVATIVES SELECTED FOR CLINICAL TRIALS

The compounds which are currently in clinical trials are semisynthetic derivatives with A- and B-ring substitutions (Figure 1). Topotecan is 9-(dimethylamino)methyl-10-hydroxycamptothecin[40] and CPT-11 is 7-ethyl-10-[4-(1-piperidino)-1-piperidino]-carbonyloxy-camptothecin,[41] and both are water-soluble. CPT-11 is poorly active *in vitro* but is a pro-drug for 7-ethyl-10-hydroxy-camptothecin (SN-38) (Figure 1) which is more potent than camptothecin[42,43] (Tanizawa and Pommier, manuscript in preparation). 9-aminocamptothecin (Figure 1), despite its poor water solubility, is currently in clinical trials because of its potency in human tumor xenografts.[3]

10,11-methylenedioxycamptothecin (Figure 1) is one of the most active among the 30 compounds that we have tested so far, with a potency ratio close to 10 when compared to natural camptothecin.[35,44-46] However, this derivative is not currently used in cancer chemotherapy because it has to be made by total synthesis and is poorly water-soluble.

II. RESULTS AND DISCUSSION

A. MECHANISMS OF CAMPTOTHECIN INDUCTION OF TOPO I-LINKED DNA BREAKS

In the presence of purified topo I, camptothecin induces DNA single-strand breaks,[47-51] which are coupled with DNA-protein crosslinks that correspond to the covalent linkage of topo I to the 3′ DNA termini.[34,52] There is good evidence that camptothecin stabilizes topo I-linked DNA breaks by preventing their religation.[50,53] Comparison of the DNA sequence location of camptothecin-induced and endogenous topo I cleavage sites demonstrates that (1) most (if not all) sites observed in the presence of camptothecin also occur, albeit at lower intensity, in the absence of drug, and (2) the degree of intensification produced by camptothecin differs among different sites.[48,49,51,54,55]

Topo I cleavage is strongly influenced by the local DNA base sequence. Both in the absence of drug and in the presence of camptothecin, approximately 90% of topo I sites have a T at the 3′ terminus of the breaks (position −1) where the enzyme is covalently linked to the DNA.[48-50] By contrast, position (+1) does not show significant preference in the absence of drug, while in the presence of camptothecin, G is strongly preferred.[48-50] The requirement for G(+1) has suggested that camptothecin interacts with the base at the 5′-terminus of topo I-induced DNA breaks and that the planar multi-ring system of camptothecin binds by stacking preferentially with G.[49] Such a stacking model is attractive because it is consistent with one we recently proposed for topo II inhibitors.[56-58]

In drug-treated cells, topo I-linked DNA breaks induced by camptothecins are rapidly resealed after drug removal,[29,35] which implies that camptothecin binding to the topo

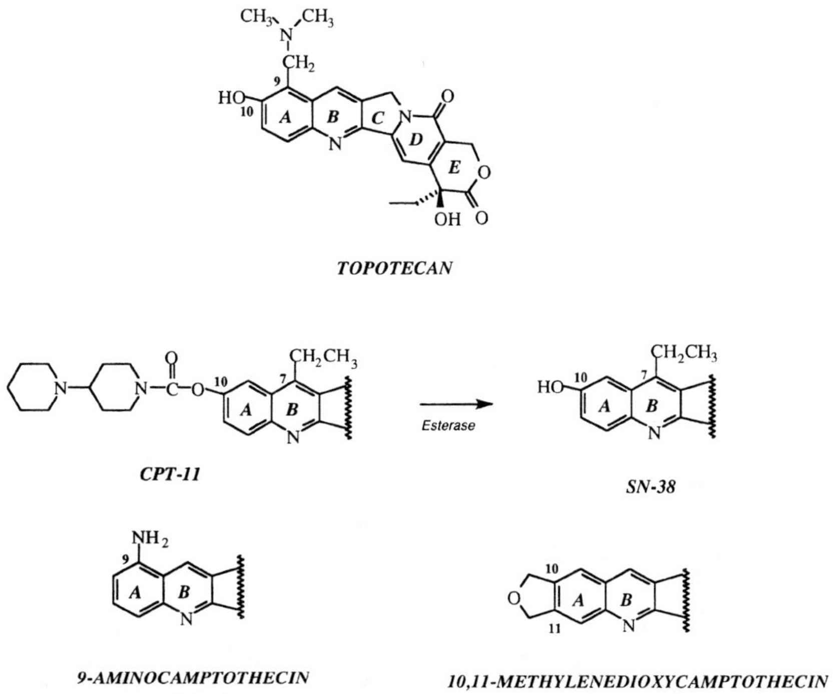

TOPOTECAN

CPT-11

SN-38

9-AMINOCAMPTOTHECIN

10,11-METHYLENEDIOXYCAMPTOTHECIN

Figure 1 Structure of some camptothecin derivatives.

I-DNA complexes is readily reversible. Also, the breaks probably correspond to potentially lethal DNA damage, and further processing appears to be necessary for cell killing. Indeed, calcium chelation or DNA synthesis inhibition by addition of EDTA[59] or aphidicolin,[60,61] respectively, to the culture medium abrogate cytotoxicity, even though the frequency of camptothecin-induced DNA breaks is unaffected.

B. MECHANISMS OF CAMPTOTHECIN CYTOTOXICITY

Camptothecin cytotoxicity is highly dependent upon the duration of the exposure to the drug.[60] This is consistent with cytotoxicity confined to certain phases of the cell cycle and is in accord with early studies showing that camptothecin is only toxic against proliferating cells.[62-64] Because topo I is present throughout the cell cycle,[5-7] however, the limited cell killing could not be attributed to variations in topo I content.

As mentioned above, the results with the DNA synthesis inhibitors, aphidicolin and hydroxyurea, indicate that lethal lesions seem to be generated by collision of active replication forks with camptothecin-trapped topo I-DNA cleavage complexes (Figure 2).[60,61] This may in part explain the recent observation that simultaneous association of camptothecin with topo II inhibitors produces antagonism not attributable to reduced formation or alterations in the rates of cleavable complex formation and reversal.[65-67] Rather, protection correlates with the kinetics of DNA and RNA synthesis inhibition produced by either drug. The antagonism between topo II inhibitors and camptothecin occurs only when the two drugs are administered simultaneously.[65]

The collision model implies that only those camptothecin-induced topo I-linked DNA breaks occurring within genomic regions being replicated at that time would be lethal. At the collison site, it is possible that DNA polymerase dissociates from the 5′-OH termini of the topo I-mediated DNA breaks and that this process generates DNA double-strand

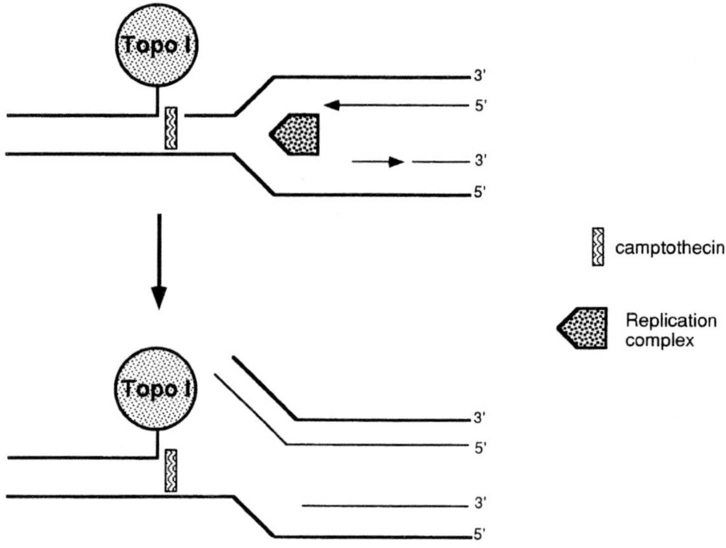

Figure 2 DNA damage induced by DNA replication through a camptothecin-stabilized cleavable complex.

breaks in newly replicated DNA. Such lesions have been identified in replicating SV40 DNA[68-71] and in genomic DNA by pulse-field gel electrophoresis.[72] This type of DNA lesion may be difficult for the cell to repair; which may explain why DNA replication inhibition is only partially reversible after camptothecin removal, while topo I-induced DNA single-strand breaks reverse very quickly.[35,45,60,63,73]

Depending on the cell type and the extent of camptothecin-induced topo I-linked DNA breaks, DNA double-strand breaks may kill cells rapidly during S-phase by apoptosis (human promyelocytic HL-60 cells),[74,75] or elicit a G_2 block.[75-77] The latter may allow DNA repair and favor cell survival (Figure 3).

C. GENERAL RESISTANCE MECHANISMS TO CAMPTOTHECIN

Figure 3 outlines the main cellular determinants of sensitivity and resistance.

Camptothecin, 9-aminocamptothecin, and probably CPT-11 are not substrate of the P-glycoprotein multi drug-resistant transporter. By contrast, recent evidence suggests that topotecan activity is reduced in cells overexpressing the P-glycoprotein, albeit this reduction is small relative to the changes in doxorubicin and etoposide uptake and cytotoxicity in the same cell lines.[78-80]

By contrast to the other camptothecins, CPT-11 may be considered as a pro-drug since it has no significant inhibitory activity against purified topo I and must be hydrolyzed to SN-38 to be active. Decreased conversion of CPT-11 to SN-38 has been reported in some resistant cell lines[81] However, since most of the CPT-11 conversion probably takes place before delivery to the tumor, the relevance of such a mechanism in CPT-11 resistance remains to be determined.

As in the case of topo II, the greater the cellular levels of topo I enzyme, the greater the number of topo I-linked DNA single-strand breaks, and the greater the probability of cell death. Decreased levels of topo I appear to play a prominent role in camptothecin resistance; qualitative alterations of topo I represent another mechanism of resistance (see Table 1 and next section).

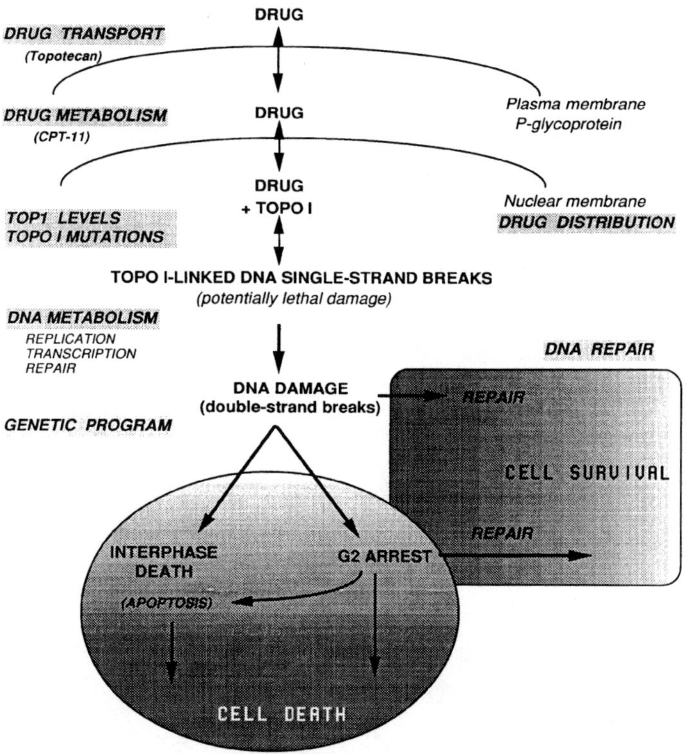

Figure 3 Determinants of sensitivity and resistance to camptothecin derivatives.

The topo I-linked DNA breaks are potentially lethal lesions and their conversion to lethal damage depends upon their interference with DNA replication (see above). Nevertheless, it is interesting to mention that neither the fraction of cells in S-phase[45] nor cell doubling-time in the 60 cell lines of the NCI Drug Screening Program are well correlated with camptothecin sensitivity (Goldwasser, Kohn, and Pommier, unpublished).

Since the lethal lesions induced by camptothecin appear to be DNA double-strand breaks, it is likely that DNA repair proficiency could be essential for cell survival and drug resistance (Figure 3). Consistent with this possibility is the observation that yeast cells which are naturally resistant to camptotecin become sensitive when they bear a mutated RAD52 gene which is essential for DNA double-strand break repair.[36,38]

D. OVERVIEW OF THE CAMPTOTHECIN-RESISTANT CELL LINES

In order to elucidate the mechanism of acquisition of resistance to CPT, several cell lines resistant to the drug have been established and analyzed (Table 1). At the dawn of camptothecin investigation, Kessel[82] first reported the pioneering work of establishment and characterization of camptothecin-resistant line of a murine leukemia, L1210/CN, by serial passage of the cells through mice in the presence of the drug. Not much characterization was performed except the one in which no increase in life span (ILS) was obtained in mice inoculated with the resistant cells and treated with the drug, while 200% of ILS was obtained in mice inoculated with parental cells and similarly treated with camptothecin.

Table 1 **Characteristics of CPT-resistant cell lines**

Cell Line	Selecting Agent	Origin	RI	Topo I Level	CPT-Sensitivity of Topo I	Topo I Gene Alteration	Ref.
				In Vitro **Mutagenesis and/or Adaptation**			
CPT-K5	CPT-11	Human T-cell ALL	300	0.3–0.5	R	Base change mutation	Andoh et al.[83-87]
PC-7/CPT	CPT-11	Human NSC lung cancer	9	0.25	R	Base change mutation	Kanzawa et al.[81,93]
HT-29/CPT	CPT	Human colon cancer	7	0.13	S	Deletion in one allele	Sugimoto et al.[88]
A549/CPT	CPT	Human lung cancer	2	1.0	ND	ND	
St-4/CPT	CPT	Human gastric cancer	9	0.25	ND	ND	
Cpt^R-B	CPT	Chinese hamster ovary (CHO)	250–350	0.4–0.5	R	ND	Gupta et al.[91]
DC3F/C-10	CPT	Chinese hamster lung (CHL)	134	1.0	R	Base change mutation	Tanizawa and Pommier[89,92]
V79^r	CPT	Chinese hamster lung (CHL)	14	0.25	ND		Change et al.[90]
IRS-1^r	CPT	CHL	2	1.0	S	cell. uptake low	
IRS-2^r	CPT	CHL	34	0.5	R	cell. uptake low	
				In Vivo **Adaptation**			
L1210/CN	CPT	Murine leukemia	ND	ND	ND	ND	Kessel[82] No ILS on CPT administration *in vivo*
P388/CPT	CPT-11	Murine leukemia	45	0.3	ND	ND	Sugimoto et al.[88]
P388/CPT	CPT	Murine leukemia	8	0.25–0.5	S	Rearrangement in one allele	Tan et al.[94]; Eng et al.[95]

RI = Resistance index; R = resistant; S = sensitive; ND = not determined.

Since the revival of the drug in the 1980s as less toxic derivatives such as CPT-11, topotecan, etc. and the discovery of topo I being the target of the drug, attention was again focused on the drug resistance. In 1987 Okada and his colleagues established and characterized a camptothecin-resistant cell line, CPT-K5, from human T-ALL RPMI8402 cells,[83-87] fuller account of which will follow. Since then, several cell lines resistant to camptothecin have been established by different methods that have generated broad cellular resistance phenotypes. The characteristics of all these resistant cell lines are summarized in Table 1. Resistance indices vary from 2 to 300-fold; topo I level is generally reduced to 0.13–0.5 except in a few cell lines, A549/CPT,[88] DC3F/C-10,[89] and IRS-1^r.[90] In several cell lines, CPT-K5,[83,84] Cpt^R-B,[91] PC-7/CPT,[81] DC3F/C-10,[89] and IRS-2^r,[90] topo I has been shown to be qualitatively altered such that the activity is resistant to the drug. Genetic alteration in the topo I gene has been demonstrated in several cell lines: base change-type mutations were shown in CPT-K5,[86] DC3F/C-10,[92] and in PC-7/CPT,[93] deletion in one allele in HT-29/CPT (Tsukahara, S., Sugimoto, Y., and Tsuruo, manuscript in preparation), and rearrangement in one allele in P388/CPT.[94,95] These cell lines seem to have acquired camptothecin-resistance by different mechanisms: (1) qualitative alteration of topo I becoming resistant to camptothecin as in CPT-K5, DC3F/C-10, Cpt^R-B, PC-7/CPT, and IRS-2^r; (2) quantitative reduction of topo I of the wild-type as in HT-29/CPT and P388/CPT; (3) reduction of cellular uptake of camptothecin as in IRS-1^r and IRS-2^r; (4) mixed type as in IRS-2^r. It is of particular interest to note that, as shown in IRS-1^r and IRS-2^r, cells appeared to develop some sort of resistance for camptothecin uptake independent of MDR-1, since camptothecin but not topotecan was shown to escape the efflux by MDR-1.[79,80,96]

Some of the camptothecin-resistant cell lines such as CPT-K5, Cpt^r-B, HT-29/CPT, St-4/CPT, P388/CPT, V79^r, and IRS-2^r show 3- to 5-fold enhanced sensitivity, i.e., collateral sensitivity, toward various drugs that inhibit topo II, i.e., teniposide, etoposide, doxorubicin, mitoxantrone, amsacrine, and ellipticine. It is conceivable that the decrease and/or some alteration in topo I activity may result in an increased reliance on limited amount of topo II for cellular function. More topo II activity may be required for cells to function in topo I-altered cells. This phenomenon could result in hypersensitivity to topo II inhibitors. Further analyses of these cell lines are needed for the elucidation of camptothecin resistance.

E. TOPO I MUTATIONS IN HUMAN CPT-K5 CELLS

Topo I from CPT-K5 Cells Has Some Altered Properties. As discussed above, topo I cleavage is strongly influenced by local DNA base sequence. Several types of cleavage sites have been identified by using camptothecin mapping studies.[54] Class A includes cleavage sites that are only slightly affected by camptothecin. Class B sites are characterized by a high degree of cleavage enhancement due to the drug action. Topo I from CPT-K5 cells exhibits some altered properties in addition to a high degree of camptothecin resistance. Camptothecin enhances the kinetic stability of the cleavable complex formed by the wild-type enzyme at a preferred topo I recognition sequence (class A site), whereas that of the mutant enzyme is not affected.[54,84] Utilizing a newly developed method of "foreign religation", the mutant enzyme was demonstrated to bind with higher affinity to and perform the catalytic reaction with higher efficiency at the camptothecin-enhanced cleavage sites (class B sites) which are otherwise not shown up by the mutant enzyme.[97] This higher activity is the result of improved DNA binding to this site and change of equilibrium between cleavage and religation being shifted toward the religation step with the mutant enzyme. The mutant topo I appears to have lost the absolute requirement of divalent cations for cleavage, while the wild-type enzyme requires them.[84] Despite the differences in enzymatic properties, the mutant enzyme was shown to perform required function in an *in vitro* system for SV40 DNA replication.[87] Thus, the mutant topo I shares similar sequence specificity with the wild-type topo I but possesses altered enzymatic properties. This enhanced DNA binding and catalysis by the mutant enzyme at the "concealed" class B sites is likely to be the basis of the camptothecin resistance of the enzyme.

Determination of Mutation Sites in CPT-K5 Topo I by cDNA Cloning and Nucleotide Sequencing. cDNA clones were isolated from cDNA libraries constructed in λgt11 vector from both cell lines. Nucleotide sequences of the clones were determined and the amino acid sequences deduced. Comparison of the sequences of the wild-type and CPT-K5 cDNAs revealed two nucleotide substitutions changing Asp-533 (GAC) and Asp-583 (GAC) of the wild-type topo I to Gly (GGC), i.e., D533G and D583G, at both sites[86] (Figure 3).

A question arises as to which mutation is responsible for camptothecin resistance of CPT-K5 topo I. Both mutation sites are in the regions where amino acid sequences are well conserved among eukaryotic topo I.[98] It is particularly notable that the amino acid residues corresponding to position 533 of the wild-type topo I are aspartic acid in all species compared including the one from mouse,[99] with the exception of glycine in CPT-K5 topo I, whereas the residues corresponding to the second site at 583 are variable, i.e., aspartic acid in the parental wild-type and human brain stem cell topo I, and glycine in all other species compared. This suggests that the differences at 583 (Asp or Gly) among the human enzymes are the result of a polymorphism of the genome unrelated to camptothecin resistance and that the key mutation responsible for the resistance is D533G. To determine this issue, enzymes with single mutation were created by site-directed mutagenesis and expression in *E. coli*.

Site-Directed Mutagenesis Determined D533G Mutation Responsible for CPT Resistance. We have constructed a series of plasmids containing inserts of topo I cDNA, corresponding to amino acid residues 163–765, with a single mutation at either 533 or 583 which was created by *in vitro* mutagenesis and as a fusion protein with glutathione-S-transferase (GST). The recombinant enzymes produced in *E. coli* were partially purified by GST-Sepharose, digested with Factor Xa to release free topo I, and assayed for the sensitivity to camptothecin. Relaxation activity of the fusion proteins of the parental type, i.e., -D-D-, at 533 and 583, and that with a single mutation at 583, i.e., -D-G-, were inhibited by camptothecin at 1 u*M* or higher concentrations, whereas that of the fusion protein with CPT-K5 type, i.e., -G-G, were not affected by camptothecin at concentrations up to 125 uM, resistance index of the latter two enzymes being more than 125. These results establish that the single mutation D533G is, in fact, responsible for the camptothecin resistance.[100]

F. TOPO I MUTATIONS IN THE CHINESE HAMSTER DC3F/C-10 CELLS

Topo I from DC3F/C-10 Cells Has Altered Properties. DC3F/C-10 cells are also highly resistant to camptothecin (Table 1). The following biochemical data strongly suggest qualitative alteration of topo I in DC3F/C-10 cells.[89] Cell lysates and nuclear extracts from DC3F/C-10 cells do not have reduced amounts of immunoreactive 100 kDa topo I protein, as detected with human scleroderma serum, when compared to those from parental DC3F cells. However, alkaline elution showed that DC3F/C-10 cells and isolated nuclei produce markedly less DNA single-strand breaks after 30 min treatment of camptothecin than DC3F cells. Northern blot analysis revealed that the amount of topo I mRNA from DC3F/C-10 cells is greater than that from DC3F cells and showed no size difference between the messages from both cell lines. Actually, purified topo I from DC3F/C-10 cells has the same molecular weight as that from DC3F cells indicating no gross difference between DC3F/C-10 and DC3F topo I enzymes. Therefore, neither quantitative reduction of topo I nor decreased cellular uptake of camptothecin seem responsible for camptothecin resistance but rather, qualitative alteration of topo I.

DNA relaxation assays revealed that the specific activity of purified 100-kDa topo I from DC3F/C-10 cells is approximately 5-fold lower than that from DC3F cells. Reduction of specific activity is a unique characteristic of DC3F/C-10 cells when compared to other CPT-resistant cell lines (Table 1). Catalytic activity of DC3F/C-10 topo I is not effectively inhibited by 10 μM camptothecin, while the same camptothecin concentration inhibits approximately 92% of the catalytic activity of DC3F topo I. Using the Fok I fragment of SV40 DNA which contains a strong camptothecin-inducible topo I cleavage site,[48,49] purified enzymes from DC3F and DC3F/C-10 cells cleaved DNA at the same position in the presence of camptothecin as previously reported by Jaxel et al.[48] However, the topo I enzyme from DC3F/C-10 cells is highly resistant to campothecin-induced cleavage.[89]

Determination of a Single Mutation Site in DC3F/C-10 Topo I by cDNA Cloning and Sequencing. Since no difference is detectable between the topo I genes from DC3F and DC3F/C-10 cells by southern blot analysis, resistance to camptothecin is not due to gross rearrangement of the topo I gene. In order to identify possible mutations, cDNA libraries from DC3F and DC3F/C-10 cells were constructed with ZAP-cDNA™ synthesis kit (Stratagene) and screened with human topo I cDNA. cDNA sequences were determined by the dideoxynucleotide chain-termination method.[92]

We found that topo I cDNA from DC3F/C-10 cells codes 767 amino acids, as mouse topo I cDNA.[92,99] Comparison of topo I cDNAs from DC3F and DC3F/C-10 cells reveals a single point mutation (G to A). This mutation results in an amino acid change from Gly-505 to Ser, which corresponds to Gly-503 in human topo I cDNA (Figure 4). This Gly is conserved among all the cloned topo I cDNAs and relatively close to the mutation site in topo I from CPT-K5 cells (Asp533-Gly).[92] Moreover, there is no difference of amino acid sequence between DC3F/C-10 and human topo I except for two additional amino acids in DC3F/C-10 topo I, which has been also found in mouse topo I cDNA. Therefore, a single amino acid change (Gly-505-Ser) seems to be responsible for both reduction of catalytic activity and resistance to camptothecin of DC3F/C-10 topo I.

III. CONCLUSIONS AND PERSPECTIVES

One accepted model of inhibition of topo I by camptothecin[46,101] postulates that upon formation of a covalently linked enzyme-DNA complex, a cleavable complex, as an intermediate of the catalytic cycle, the enzyme undergoes a conformation change which produces a site or pocket fitting camptothecin, to which the drug molecule binds avidly, stabilizing the ternary complex, inhibiting the religation half-reaction, and immobilizing the enzyme from turnover. Bjornsti et al.[102] reported earlier that a mutation changing glycine to cysteine at residue 363 (G363C) in a plasmid-borne human topo I gene confers camptothecin resistance to the plasmid-transformed yeast cells. Kubota et al.[93] reported still another mutation at amino acid residue 729 in topo I changing threonine to alanine (T729A) in a camptothecin-resistant human small cell lung cancer cell line PC-7/CPT. More recently, Fujimori et al.[103] sequenced another mutation in the catalytic tyrosine (Y723) region changing asparagine to serine (N722S) in a camptothecin-resistant human leukemia cell line and demonstrated that the mutated recombinant enzyme was resistant to camptothecin.[103] Thus, the finding that the mutations occurring at different sites, i.e., G363C, D533G, N722S, and T729A in human topo I, and G505S in hamster topo I are contained in well-conserved regions, and these mutations conferring resistance to camptothecin are consistent with the hypothesis that the domains around these residues are critical for catalytic activity and interaction with camptothecin. Taken together with the stacking model for camptothecin interaction at the topo I-DNA sites (49; see above), these observations suggest a possible folding of the topo I protein bringing into proximity the central domain, where mutations have been detected, and the active tyrosine region.

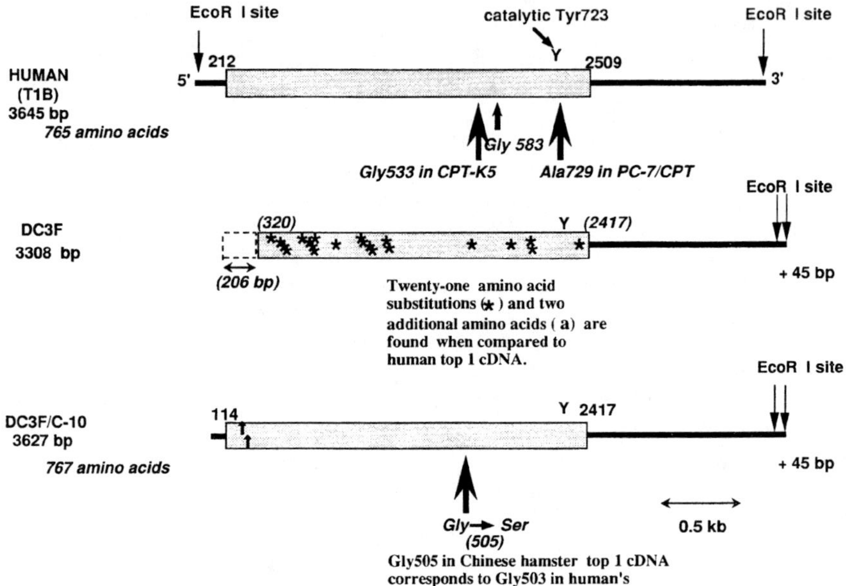

Figure 4 Schematic representation of the topo I mutations in human and Chinese hamster camptothecin-resistant cell lines. The shaded boxes correspond to the topo I cDNAs. Cell lines are indicated to the left.

ACKNOWLEDGMENTS

Y.P. wishes to thank Dr. Kurt W. Kohn for valuable discussion and support during the course of the work presented here.

REFERENCES

1. **Juan, C. C., Hwang, J. L., Liu, A. A., Whang-Peng, J., Knutsen, T., Huebner, K., Croce, C. M., Zhang, H., Wang, J. C., and Liu, L. F.,** Human DNA topoisomerase I is encoded by a single-copy gene that maps to chromosome region 20q12-13.2. *Proc. Natl. Acad. Sci. U.S.A.,* 85: 8910-8913, 1988.

2. **D'Arpa, P., Machlin, P. S., Ratrie, H., 3d, Rothfield, N. F., Cleveland, D. W., and Earnshaw, W. C.,** cDNA cloning of human DNA topoisomerase I: catalytic activity of a 67.7-kDa carboxyl-terminal fragment. *Proc. Natl. Acad. Sci. U.S.A.,* 85: 2543-2547, 1988.

3. **Giovanella, B. C., Stehlin, J. S., Wall, M. E., Wani, M. C., Nicholas, A. W., Liu, L. F., Silber, R., and Potmesil, M.,** DNA topoisomerase I-targeted chemotherapy of human colon cancer in xenografts. *Science,* 246: 1046-1048, 1989.

4. **van der Zee, A. G. J., Hollema, H., de Jong, S., Boonstra, H., Gouw, A., Willemse, P. H. B., Zijlstra, J. G., and de Vrie, E. G. E.,** P-glycoprotein expression and DNA topoisomerase I and II activity in benign tumors of the ovary and in malignant tumors of the ovary, before and after platinum/cyclophosphamide chemotherapy. *Cancer Res.,* 51: 5915-5920, 1991.

5. **Heck, M. M., Hittelman, W. N., and Earnshaw, W. C.,** Differential expression of DNA topoisomerases I and II during the eukaryotic cell cycle. *Proc. Natl. Acad. Sci. U.S.A.,* 85: 1086-1090, 1988.

6. **Romig, H. and Richter, A.,** Expression of the topoisomerase I gene in serum-stimulated human fibroblasts. *Biochim. Biophys. Acta.,* 1048: 274-280, 1990.

7. **Duguet, M., Lavenot, C., Harper, F., Mirambeau, G., and De Recondo, A. M.,** DNA topoisomerases from rat liver: physiological variations. *Nucleic Acids Res.,* 11: 1059-1075, 1983.

8. **Taudou, G., Mirambeau, G., Lavenot, C., Dergarabedian, A., Vermeersch, J., and Duguet, M.,** DNA topoisomerase activities in concanavalin A-stimulated lymphocytes. *FEBS Lett.,* 176: 431-435, 1984.

9. **Durban, E., Mills, J. S., Roll, D., and Busch, H.,** Phosphorylation of purified Novikoff hepatoma topoisomerase I. *Biochem. Biophys. Res. Commun.,* 111: 897-905, 1983.

10. **Durban, E., Goodenough, M., Mills, J., and Busch, H.,** Topoisomerase I phosphorylation *in vitro* and in rapidly growing Novikoff hepatoma cells. *Embo. J.,* 4: 2921-2926, 1985.

11. **Tse-Dinh, Y. C., Wong, T. W., and Goldberg, A. R.,** Virus- and cell-encoded tyrosine protein kinases inactivate DNA topoisomerases *in vitro. Nature,* 312: 785-786, 1984.

12. **Kaiserman, H. B., Ingebritsen, T. S., and Benbow, R. M.,** Regulation of *Xenopus laevis* DNA topoisomerase I activity by phosphorylation *in vitro. Biochemistry,* 27: 3216-3222, 1988.

13. **Samuel, D. S., Shimizu, Y., and Shimizu, N.,** Protein kinase C phosphorylates DNA topoisomerase I. *FEBS Lett.,* 259: 57-60, 1989.

14. **Pommier, Y., Kerrigan, D., Hartmann, K. D., and Glazer, R. I.,** Phosphorylation of mammalian DNA topoisomerase I and activation by protein C. *J. Biol. Chem.,* 16: 9418-9422, 1990.

15. **Coderoni, S., Paparelli, M., Luigi, G., and Gianfranceschi, G. L.,** Phosphorylation sites for type N II protein kinase in DNA-topoisomerase I from calf thymus. *Int. J. Biochem.,* 22: 737-746, 1990.

16. **Samuels, D. S. and Shimizu, N.,** DNA topoisomerase I phosphorylation in murine fibroblasts treated with 12-O-tetradecanoylphorbol-13-acetate and *in vitro* by protein kinase C. *J. Biol. Chem.,* 267: 11156-11162, 1992.

17. **Utsugi, T., Mattern, M. R., Mirabelli, C. K., and Hanna, N.,** Potentiation of topoisomerase inhibitor-induced DNA strand breakage and cytotoxicity by tumor necrosis factor: enhancement of topoisomerase activity as a mechanism of potentiation. *Cancer Res.,* 50: 2636-2640, 1990.

18. **Nambi, P., Mattern, M., Bartus, J. O. L., Aiyar, N., and Crooke, S. T.,** Stimulation of intracellular topoisomerase I activity by vasopressin and thrombin. *Biochem. J.,* 262: 485-489, 1989.

19. **Nambi, P., Wu, H.-L., Woessner, R. D., and Mattern, M. R.,** Inhibition of endothelium-mediated topoisomerase I activation by pertussis toxin. *FEBS Lett.,* 276: 17-20, 1990.

20. **Mattern, M. R., Mong, S., Mong, S.-M., Bartus, J., Sarau, H. M., Clark, M. A., Foley, J. J., and Crooke, S. T.,** Transient activation of topoisomerase I in leukotriene D4 signal transduction in human cells. *Biochem. J.,* 265: 101-107, 1990.

21. **Jongstra-Bilen, J., Ittel, M. E., Niedergang, C., Vosberg, H. P., and Mandel, P.,** DNA topoisomerase I from calf thymus is inhibited *in vitro* by poly(ADP-ribosylation). *Eur. J. Biochem.,* 136: 391-396, 1983.

22. **Ferro, A. M., Higgins, N. P., and Olivera, B. M.,** Poly (ADP-ribosylation) of a DNA topoisomerase. *J. Biol. Chem.,* 258: 6000-6003, 1983.

23. **Ferro, A. M., McElwain, M. C., and Olivera, B. M.,** Poly(ADP-ribosylation) of DNA topoisomerase I: a nuclear response to DNA-strand interruptions. *Cold Spring Harb. Symp. Quant. Biol.,* 49: 683-690, 1984.

24. **Ferro, A. M., Thompson, L. H., and Olivera, B. M.,** Poly (ADP-ribosylation) and DNA topoisomerase I in different cell lines. *Adv. Exp. Med. Biol.,* 179: 441-447, 1984.

25. **Ferro, A. M., and Olivera, B. M.,** Poly(ADP-ribosylation) of DNA topoisomerase I from calf thymus. *J. Biol. Chem.,* 259: 547-554, 1984.

26. **Darby, M. K., Schmitt, B., Jongstra-Bilen, J., and Vosberg, H. P.,** Inhibition of calf thymus type II DNA topoisomerase by poly(ADP-ribosylation). *Embo. J.,* 4: 2129-2134, 1985.

27. **Kasid, U. N., Halligan, B., Liu, L. F., Dritschilo, A., and Smulson, M.,** Poly(ADP-ribose)-mediated post-translational modification of chromatin-associated human topoisomerase I. Inhibitory effects on catalytic activity. *J. Biol. Chem.,* 264: 18687-18692, 1989.

28. **Krupita, G. and Cerutti, P.,** ADP-ribosylation of ADPR-transferase and topoisomerase I in intact mouse epidermal cell JB6. *Biochemistry,* 28: 2034-2040, 1989.

29. **Mattern, M. R., Mong, S. M., Bartus, H. F., Mirabelli, C. K., Crooke, S. T., and Johnson, R. K.,** Relationship between the intracellular effects of camptothecin and the inhibition of DNA topoisomerase I in cultured L1210 cells. *Cancer Res.,* 47: 1793-1798, 1987.

30. **Tamura, H.-O., Ikegami, Y., Ono, K., Sekimizu, K., and Andoh, T.,** Acidic phospholipids directly inhibit DNA binding of mammalian DNA topoisomerase I. *FEBS Lett.,* 261: 151-154, 1990.

31. **Ishii, K., Katase, A., Andoh, T., and Seno, N.,** Inhibition of topoisomerase I by heparine. *Biochem. Biophys. Res. Commun.,* 104: 541-547, 1987.

32. **Jaxel, C., Kohn, K. W., Wani, M. C., Wall, M. E., and Pommier, Y.,** Structure-activity study of the actions of camptothecin derivatives on mammalian topoisomerase I: evidence for a specific receptor site and a relation to antitumor activity. *Cancer Res.,* 49: 1465-1469, 1989.

33. **Nicholas, A. W., Wani, M. C., Manikumar, G., Wall, M. E., Kohn, K. W., and Pommier, Y.,** Plant antitumor agents. 29. Synthesis and biological activity of ring D and ring E modified analogues of camptothecin. *J. Med. Chem.,* 33: 972-978, 1990.

34. **Hsiang, Y. H. and Liu, L. F.,** Identification of mammalian DNA topoisomerase I as an intracellular target of the anticancer drug camptothecin. *Cancer Res.,* 48: 1722-1726, 1988.

35. **Covey, J. M., Jaxel, C., Kohn, K. W., and Pommier, Y.,** Protein-linked DNA strand breaks induced in mammalian cells by camptothecin, an inhibitor of topoisomerase I. *Cancer Res.,* 49: 5016-5022, 1989.

36. **Nitiss, J. and Wang, J. C.,** DNA topoisomerase-targeting antitumor drugs can be studied in yeast. *Proc. Natl. Acad. Sci. U.S.A.,* 85: 7501-7505, 1988.

37. **Bjornsti, M.-A., Benedetti, P., Viglianti, G. A., and Wang, J. C.,** Expression of human DNA topoisomerase I in yeast cells lacking yeast DNA topoisomerase I: restoration of sensitivity of the cells to the antitumor drug camptothecin. *Cancer Res.,* 49: 6318-6323, 1989.

38. **Eng, W. K., Faucette, L., Johnson, R. K., and Sternglanz, R.,** Evidence that DNA topoisomerase I is necessary for the cytotoxic effects of camptothecin. *Mol. Pharmacol.,* 34: 755-760, 1988.

39. **Madden, K. R., and Champoux, J. J.,** Overexpression of human topoisomerase I in baby hamster kidney cells: hypersensitivity of clonal isolates to camptothecin. *Cancer Res.,* 52: 525-532, 1992.

40. **Johnson, R. K., McCabe, F. L., Faucette, L. F., Hertzberg, R. P., Kingsbury, W. D., Boehm, J. C., Caranfa, M. J., and Holden, K. G.,** SK&F 10864, a water-soluble analog of camptothecin with broad-spectrum activity in preclinical tumor models. *Proc. Am. Assoc. Cancer Res.,* 30: 623, 1989.

41. **Kunimoto, T., Nitta, K., Tanaka, T., Uebuara, N., Baba, H., Takeuchi, M., Yokokura, T., Sawada, S., Miyasaka, T., and Mutai, M.,** Antitumor activity of 7-ethyl-10-[4-(1-piperidino)-1-piperidino]carbonyloxy-camptothecin, a novel water-soluble derivative of camptothecin, against murine tumors. *Cancer Res.,* 47: 5944-5947, 1987.

42. **Kaneda, N., Nagata, H., Furuta, T., and Yokokura, T.,** Metabolism and pharmacokinetics of the camptothecin analogue CPT-11 in the mouse. *Cancer Res.,* 50: 1715-1720, 1990.

43. **Kawato, Y., Aonuma, M., Hirota, Y., Kuga, H., and Sato, K.,** Intracellular roles of SN-38, a metabolite of the camptothecin derivative CPT-11, in the antitumor effect of CPT-11. *Cancer Res.,* 51: 4187-4191, 1991.

44. **O'Connor, P. M., Kerrigan, D., Bertrand, R., Kohn, K. W., and Pommier, Y.,** 10,11-methylenedioxycamptothecin, a topoisomerase I inhibitor of increased potency: DNA damage and correlation to cytotoxicity in human colon carcinoma (HT-29) cells. *Cancer Comm.,* 2: 395-400, 1990.

45. **O'Connor, P. M., Nieves-Neira, W., Kerrigan, D., Bertrand, R., Goldman, J., Kohn, K. W., and Pommier, Y.,** S-Phase population analysis does not correlate with the cytotoxicity of camptothecin and 10,11-methylenedioxycamptothecin in human colon carcinoma HT-29 cells. *Cancer Comm.,* 3: 233-240, 1991.

46. **Pommier, Y., Jaxel, C., Kerrigan, D., and Kohn, K. W.,** Structure activity relationship of topoisomerase I inhibition by camptothecin derivatives: evidence for the existence of a ternary complex. In Potmesil, M. and Kohn, K. W., Eds., *DNA Topoisomerases in Cancer,* Oxford University Press, New York, 1991, 121-132.

47. **Hsiang, Y. H., Hertzberg, R., Hecht, S., and Liu, L. F.,** Camptothecin induces protein-linked DNA breaks via mammalian DNA topoisomerase I. *J. Biol. Chem.,* 260: 14873-14878, 1985.

48. **Jaxel, C., Kohn, K. W., and Pommier, Y.,** Topoisomerase I interaction with SV40 DNA in the presence and absence of camptothecin. *Nucleic Acids Res.,* 16: 11157-11170, 1988.

49. **Jaxel, C., Capranico, G., Kerrigan, D., Kohn, K. W., and Pommier, Y.,** Effect of local DNA sequence on topoisomerase I cleavage in the presence or absence of camptothecin. *J. Biol. Chem.,* 266: 20418-20423, 1991.

50. **Porter, S. E., and Champoux, J. J.,** The basis for camptothecin enhancement of DNA breakage by eukaryotic topoisomerase I. *Nucleic Acids Res.,* 17: 8521-8532, 1989.

51. **Thomsen, B., Mollerup, S., Bonven, B. J., Frank, R., Blocker, H., Nielsen, O. F., and Westergaard, O.,** Sequence specificity of DNA topoisomerase I in the presence and absence of camptothecin. *Embo. J.,* 6: 1817-1823, 1987.

52. **Champoux, J. J.,** Mechanism of the reaction catalyzed by the DNA untwisting enzyme: attachment of the enzyme to 3'-terminus of the nicked DNA. *J. Mol. Biol.,* 118: 441-446, 1978.

53. **Svejstrup, J. Q., Christiansen, K., Gromova, I. I., Andersen, A. H., and Westergaard, O.,** New technique for uncoupling the cleavage and religation reactions of eukaryotic topoisomerase I. The mode of action of camptothecin at a specific recognition site. *J. Mol. Biol.,* 222: 669-678, 1991.

54. **Kjeldsen, E., Mollerup, S., Thomsen, B., Bonven, B. J., Bolund, L., and Westergaard, O.,** Sequence-dependent effect of camptothecin on human topoisomerase I DNA cleavage. *J. Mol. Biol.,* 202: 333-342, 1988.

55. **Porter, S. E. and Champoux, J. J.,** Mapping *in vivo* topoisomerase I sites on simian virus 40 DNA: asymmetric distribution of sites on replicating molecules. *Mol. Cell. Biol.,* 9: 541-550, 1989.

56. **Capranico, G., Kohn, K. W., and Pommier, Y.,** Local sequence requirements for DNA cleavage by mammalian topoisomerase II in the presence of doxorubicin. *Nucleic Acids Res.,* 18: 6611-6619, 1990.

57. **Pommier, Y., Capranico, G., Orr, A., and Kohn, K. W.,** Local base sequence preferences for DNA cleavage by mammalian topoisomerase II in the presence of amsacrine and teniposide. *Nucleic Acids Res.,* 19: 5973-5980, 1991.

58. **Pommier, Y. and Tanizawa, A.,** DNA topoisomerase I and its inhibitors. In Tritton, T. R. and Hickman, J. A., Eds., *Cancer Chemotherapy,* Blackwell, London, 1992.

59. **Bertrand, R., Kerrigan, D., Sarang, M., and Pommier, Y.,** Cell death induced by topoisomerase inhibitors: role of calcium in mammalian cells. *Biochem. Pharmacol.,* 42: 77-85, 1991.

60. **Holm, C., Covey, J. M., Kerrigan, D., and Pommier, Y.,** Differential requirement of DNA replication for the cytotoxicity of DNA topoisomerase I and II inhibitors in Chinese hamster DC3F cells. *Cancer Res.,* 49: 6365-6368, 1989.

61. **Hsiang, Y.-H., Lihou, M. G., and Liu, L. F.,** Arrest of DNA replication by drug-stabilized topoisomerase I-DNA cleavable complexes as a mechanism of cell killing by camptothecin. *Cancer Res.,* 49: 5077-5082, 1989.

62. **Horwitz, S. B. and Horwitz, M. S.,** Effects of camptothecin on the breakage and repair of DNA during the cell cycle. *Cancer Res.,* 33: 2834-2836, 1973.

63. **Kessel, D., Bosmann, H. B., and Lohr, K.,** Camptothecin effects on DNA synthesis in murine leukemia cells. *Biochim. Biophys. Acta.,* 269: 210-216, 1972.

64. **Li, L. H., Fraser, T. J., Olin, E. J., and Bhuyan, B. K.,** Action of camptothecin on mammalian cells in culture. *Cancer Res.,* 32: 2643-2650, 1972.

65. **Bertrand, R., O'Connor, P., Kerrigan, D., and Pommier, Y.,** Sequential administration of camptothecin and etoposide circumvents the antagonistic cytotoxicity of simultaneous drug administration in slowly growing human carcinoma, HT-29 cells. *Eur. J. Cancer,* 28A: 743-748, 1992.

66. **D'Arpa, P., Beardmore, C., and Liu, L. F.,** Involvement of nucleic acid synthesis in cell killing mechanisms of topoisomerase poisons. *Cancer Res.,* 50: 6919-6924, 1990.

67. **Kaufmann, S. H.,** Antagonism between camptothecin and topoisomerase II-directed chemotherapeutic agents in a human leukemia cell line. *Cancer Res.,* 51: 1129-1136, 1991.

68. **Avemann, K., Knippers, R., Koller, T., and Sogo, J. M.,** Camptothecin, a specific inhibitor of type I DNA topoisomerase, induces DNA breakage at replication forks. *Mol. Cell. Biol.,* 8: 3026-3034, 1988.

69. **Yang, L., Wold, M. S., Li, J. J., Kelly, T. J., and Liu, L. F.,** Roles of DNA topoisomerases in simian virus 40 DNA replication *in vitro. Proc. Natl. Acad. Sci. U.S.A.,* 84: 950-954, 1987.

70. **Fleischmann, G., Filipski, R., and Elgin, S. C.,** Isolation and distribution of a Drosophila protein preferentially associated with inactive regions of the genome. *Chromosoma.,* 96: 83-90, 1987.

71. **Shin, C.-G. and Snapka, R. M.,** Exposure to camptothecin breaks leading and lagging strand simian virus 40 DNA replication forks. *Biochem. Biophys. Res. Comm.,* 168: 135-140, 1990.

72. **Ryan, A. J., Squires, S., Strutt, H. L., and Johnson, R. T.,** Camptothecin cytotoxicity in mammalian cells is associated with the induction of persistent double-strand breaks in replicating DNA. *Nucleic Acids Res.,* 19: 3295-3300, 1991.

73. **Horwitz, S. B., Chang, C. K., and Grollman, A. P.,** Studies on camptothecin. I. Effects of nucleic acid and protein synthesis. *Mol. Pharmacol.,* 7: 632-644, 1971.

74. **Kaufmann, S. H.,** Induction of endonucleolytic DNA cleavage in human acute myelogenous leukemia cells by etoposide, camptothecin, and other cytotoxic anticancer drugs: a cautionary note. *Cancer Res.,* 49: 5870-5878, 1989.

75. **Del Bino, G., Skierski, J. S., and Darzynkiewicz, Z.,** Diverse effects of camptothecin, an inhibitor of topoisomerase I, on the cell cycle of lymphocytic (L1210, MOLT-4) and myelogenous (HL-60, KG1) leukemic cells. *Cancer Res.,* 50: 5746-5750, 1990.

76. **Tobey, R. A.,** Effects of cytosine arabinoside, daunomycin, mithramycin, azacytidine, adriamycin, and camptothecin on mammalian cell cycle traverse. *Cancer Res.,* 32: 2720-2725, 1972.

77. **Tsao, Y.-P., D'Arpa, P., and Liu, L. F.,** The involvement of active DNA synthesis in camptothecin-induced G2 arrest: altered regulation of p34cdc2/cyclin B. *Cancer Res.,* 52: 1823-1829, 1992.

78. **Naito, M., Hamada, H., and Tsuruo, T.,** ATP/Mg2+-dependent binding of vincristine to the plasma membrane of multidrug-resistant K562 cells. *J. Biol. Chem.,* 263: 11887-11891, 1988.

79. **Chen, A. Y., Yu, C., Potmesil, M., Wall, M. E., Wani, M. C., and Liu, L. F.,** Camptothecin overcomes MDR1-mediated resistance in human KB carcinoma cells. *Cancer Res.,* 51: 6039-6044, 1991.

80. **Hendricks, C. B., Rowinsky, E. K., Grochow, L. B., Donchower, R. C., and Kaufmann, S. H.,** Effect of P-glycoprotein expression on the accumulation and cytotoxicity of topotecan (SK&F 104864), a new camptothecin analogue. *Cancer Res.,* 52: 2268-2278, 1992.

81. **Kanzawa, F., Sugimoto, Y., Minato, K., Kasahara, K., Bungo, M., Nakagawa, K., Fujiwara, Y., Liu, L. F., and Saijo, N.,** Establishment of a camptothecin analogue (CPT-11)-resistant cell line of human non-small cell lung cancer: characterization and mechanism of resistance. *Cancer Res.,* 50: 5919-5924, 1990.

82. **Kessel, D.,** Some determinants of camptothecin responsiveness in leukemia L1210 cells. *Cancer Res.,* 31: 1883-1887, 1971.

83. **Andoh, T., Ishii, K., Suzuki, Y., Ikegami, Y., Kusunki, Y., Takemoto, Y., and Okada, K.,** Characterization of a mammalian mutant with a camptothecin-resistant DNA topoisomerase I. *Proc. Natl. Acad. Sci. U.S.A.,* 84: 5565-5569, 1987.

84. **Kjeldsen, E., Bonven, B. J., Andoh, T., Ishii, K., Okada, K., Bolund, L., and Westergaard, O.,** Characterization of a camptothecin-resistant human DNA topoisomerase I. *J. Biol. Chem.,* 263: 3912-3916, 1988.

85. **Oguro, M., Seki, Y., Okada, K., and Andoh, T.,** Collateral drug sensitivity induced in CPT-11 (a novel derivative of camptothecin)-resistant cell lines. *Biomed. & Pharmacother.,* 44: 209-216, 1990.

86. **Tamura, H.-O., Kohchi, C., Yamada, R., Ikeda, T., Koiwa, O., Patterson, E., Keene, J. D., Okada, K., Kjeldsen, E., Nishikawa, K., and Andoh, T.,** Molecular cloning of a cDNA of a camptothecin-resistant human DNA topoisomerase I and identification of mutation sites. *Nucleic Acids Res.,* 19: 69-75, 1991.

87. **Ishimi, Y., Nishizawa, M., and Andoh, T.,** Characterization of a camptothecin-resistant human DNA topoisomerase I in an *in vitro* system for simian virus 40 DNA replication. *Eur. J. Biochem.,* 202: 835-839, 1992.

88. **Sugimoto, Y., Tsukahara, S., Oh-hara, T., Isoe, T., and Tsuruo, T.,** Decreased expression of DNA topoisomerase I in camptothecin-resistant tumor cell lines as determined by a monoclonal antibody. *Cancer Res.,* 50: 6925-6930, 1990.

89. **Tanizawa, A. and Pommier, Y.,** Topoisomerase I alterations in a camptothecin-resistant cell line derived from Chinese hamster DC3F cells in culture. *Cancer Res.,* 52: 1848-1854, 1992.

90. **Chang, J.-Y., Dethlefsen, L. A., Barley, L. R., Zhou, B. S., and Cheng, Y.-C.,** Characterization of camptothecin-resistant Chinese hamster lung cells. *Biochem. Pharmacol.,* 43: 1732-1735, 1992.

91. **Gupta, R. S., Gupta, R., Eng, B., Lock, R. B., Ross, W. E., Hertzberg, R. P., Caranfa, M. J., and Johnson, R. K.,** Camptothecin-resistant mutants of Chinese hamster ovary cells containing a resistant form of topoisomerase I. *Cancer Res.,* 48: 6404-6410, 1988.

92. **Tanizawa, A., Tabuchi, A., Bertrand, R., and Pommier, Y.,** Cloning of Chinese hamster DNA topoisomerase I cDNA and identification of a single-point mutation responsible for camptothecin resistance. *J. Biol. Chem.,* 268: 25463-25468, 1993.

93. **Kubota, N., Kanzawa, F., Nishio, K., Takeda, Y., Ohmori, T., Fujiwara, Y., Terashima, Y., and Saijo, N.,** Detection of topoisomerase I gene point mutation in CPT-11 resistant lung cancer cell line. *Biochem. Biophys. Res. Comm.,* in press, 1992.

94. **Tan, K. B., Mattern, M. R., Eng, W.-K., McCabe, F. L., and Johnson, R. K.,** Nonproductive rearrangement of DNA topoisomerase I and II genes: correlation with resistance to topoisomerase inhibitors. *J. Natl. Cancer Inst.,* 81: 1732-1735, 1989.

95. **Eng, W. K., McCabe, F. L., Tan, K. B., Mattern, M. R., Hofmann, G. A., Woessner, R. D., Hertzberg, R. P., and Johnson, R. K.,** Development of a stable camptothecin-resistant subline of P388 leukemia with reduced topoisomerase I content. *Mol. Pharmacol.,* 38: 471-480, 1990.

96. **Tsuruo, T., Matsuzaki, T., Matsushita, M., Saito, H., and Yokokura, T.,** Antitumor effect of CPT-11, a new derivative of camptothecin, against pleiotropic drug-resistant tumors *in vitro* and *in vivo. Cancer Chemother. Pharmacol.,* 21: 71-74, 1988.

97. **Gromova, I. I., Kjeldsen, E., Svejstrup, J. Q., Alsner, J., Christiansen, K., and Westergaard, O.,** Characterization of an altered DNA catalysis of camptothecin-resistant eukaryotic topoisomerase I. *Nucleic Acids Res.,* 21: 593-600, 1993.

98. **Lynn, R. M., Bjornsti, M. A., Caron, P. R., and Wang, J. C.,** Peptide sequencing and site-directed mutagenesis identify tyrosine-727 as the active site tyrosine of saccharomyces cerevisiae DNA topoisomerase I. *Proc. Natl. Acad. Sci. U.S.A.,* 86: 3559-3563, 1989.

99. **Koiwa, O., Yasui, Y., Sakai, Y., Watanabe, T., Ishii, K., Yanagihara, S., and Andoh, T.,** Cloning of the mouse cDNA encoding DNA topoisomerase I and chromosomal location of the gene. *Gene.,* 125: 211-216, 1992.

100. **Andoh, T., Koiwai, O., and Okada, K.,** Molecular basis of resistance to CPT-11, specific inhibitor of DNA topoisomerase I. In Miyazaki, T., Takaku, F., and Sakuraba, K., Eds., *The Mechanisms and New Approach on Drug Resistance of Cancer Cells,* Elsevier Science Publishers B.U., Amsterdam, 1993, 95-101.

101. **Liu, L. F.,** DNA topoisomerase poisons as antitumor drugs. *Ann. Rev. Biochem.,* 58: 351-375, 1989.

102. **Benedetti, P., Tsai-Phlugfelder, M., and Wang, J. C.,** The use of yeast and yeast strains expressing human topoisomerases in the study of anticancer drugs. In Tsuruo, T., Ogawa, M., and Carter, S. K., Eds., *Drug Resistance as a Biochemical Target in Cancer Chemotherapy,* Academic Press, San Diego, CA, 1990, 121-145.

103. **Fujimori, A., Harker, W. G., Hoki, Y., Kohlhagen, G., and Pommier, Y.,** Mutation at the catalytic site of topoisomerase I in a human leukemia cell line resistant to camptothecin. *Proc. Amer. Assoc. Cancer Res.,* 35: 363, 1994.

The Perspectives

Milan Potmesil and Herbert Pinedo

Following a dormant period, basic scientists and clinical oncologists are again developing a number of promising cytostatics, with novel mechanisms of action and activity in several types of malignancies. Two groups of anticancer agents are to be mentioned in particular: camptothecin inhibitors of DNA topoisomerase I (topo I) and mitotic inhibitors taxanes. A recent symposium organized by the National Cancer Institute/European Organization for Research and Treatment of Cancer[1] focused on the camptothecins, and we will try to put presented materials into perspective. Interesting studies concerning molecular modeling are ongoing with camptothecin and other inhibitors of topo I, and these may elucidate similarities and differences in their cytotoxic mechanisms. It has become clear that such mechanisms of drug-topo I-DNA interaction may differ considerably. The studies will also help us to understand the development of resistance to camptothecins and suggest ways to its circumvention.

Laboratory studies indicate that the camptothecins, except topotecan, do overcome the classical type of multi-drug resistance associated with expression of the P-glycoprotein, product of the MDR1 gene. Laboratory data, however, also show that enhanced repair of DNA strand breaks or mutated forms of topo I result in resistance to camptothecins accompanied in some cell lines by decreased topo I expression and function. Since drug resistance is the main reason for treatment failure in cancer patients, laboratory research should be extended to clinical situations. This will require monitoring of tumor specimens, obtained before and during camptothecin-based chemotherapy, for relevant indicators of resistance such as topo I content, function, and structural changes of the topo-I gene. Although the known mechanism of camptothecin resistance relates directly to the target enzyme topo I, the role of complex array of suppressor or regulatory genes on topo I gene expression and drug resistance are also being explored. Studies of several mechanisms, e.g., the c-myc and/or c-H-ras genes and CPT-11 resistance,[2] the Bcl-2 protooncogene and CAM-induced apoptosis,[3,4] p53 gene mutations and resistance to various anticancer agents,[5,6] or the role of BCR-ABL gene in resistance to the apoptotic cell death[7] point in this direction.

It has been shown in human cancer studies in mouse xenografts and in tissue-culture assays that camptothecin cytotoxicity is greatly enhanced by a continuous as compared to a short-term (e.g., 1 h) exposure. This observation seems to be validated by results of a phase I low-dose 21-day infusion regimen q 1 month.[8] There are other ways which could achieve a prolonged drug exposure: (1) the oral route of delivery or (2) a tapered-off continuous infusion which provides for tapered-off plasma levels of camptothecin lactone, and this results in preferential cytotoxicity against cancerous cells with overexpressed topo I. At the same time, this schedule may spare normal hematopoietic and mucosal progenitors with low topo I levels. As to the route of application, interesting pharmacological data were obtained in the primates showing that the intrathecal administration of a camptothecin is well tolerated.[1] We believe that optimal routes of application and the schedule dependency of camptothecins are far from being established and that new schedules and methods of delivery should be explored.

There are four camptothecins already introduced into the clinic: CPT-11 (irinotecan), topotecan, 9-amino-20(S)-camptothecin, and 20(S)-camptothecin. Other compounds are ready on the doorstep. The topo I inhibitors show promising activity in major tumor types such as colorectal adenocarcinoma, gynecological cancers, and non-small or small cell lung cancer. The activity of CPT-11 and topotecan seems to differ to some extent, while their toxicities differ greatly. The optimal schedule of administration for CPT-11 has yet to be defined. The median toxic dose (MTD) for the weekly schedule is in the same range in studies performed in the U.S., France, and Japan, with 180 mg/m^2, 145 mg/m^2, and 125 mg/m^2, respectively. However, the MTD which was determined for a 3–4-week interval schedules varied from 250 mg/m^2 to 750 mg/m^2 in the three countries. The doses recommended for Phase II studies by the French group are 350 mg/m^2 (every three weeks), 115 mg/m^2 (weekly), and 100 mg/m^2 (daily $\times$ 3 q 3 weeks).[1]

A significant schedule-dependent toxicity of CPT-11 has been observed, with neutropenia (in q 3 weeks schedule) and diarrhea (both for weekly and daily $\times$ 3 q weeks) being the most prominent. Neutropenia shows a nadir between day 6 and 12 following drug administration, and it is schedule- and dose-dependent. However, no cumulative toxicity has been seen in subsequent cycles. Although CPT-11 is clearly active in cancer patients, its toxicity remains a matter of concern. Two types of gastrointestinal toxicity have been identified. The acute gastrointestinal toxic syndrome occurs during or immediately after the drug administration, with abdominal cramps, early diarrhea, diaphoresis, salivation, and lacrimation. This syndrome responds well to atropine. The late gastrointestinal toxic syndrome, consisting of severe diarrhea, is more a problem. It occurs 4–8 days after CPT-11 administration and its onset is unpredictable, with a wide interpatient and intrapatient variability. The French group has shown that diarrhea responds to some extent to high-dose Loperamide. Further studies on the mechanism of this side effect are needed to avoid a difficult management of CPT-11 treatment in the clinic. The French group selected the three-weekly schedule for Phase II trials, with the initial dose of 350 mg/m^2, which is followed by dose escalation until the MTD for individual patients has been defined. Phase II studies in Japan, on different schedules, report response rates in non-small cell lung cancer at 31.9%, in small cell lung cancer at 47%, colorectal adenocarcinoma 27%, gastric cancer 23%, and in pancreatic cancer 11%. Responses have also been observed for cancer of the uterine cervix (23%), ovarian cancer (21%), and non-Hodgkin lymphoma (49%).

The dose-limiting toxicity of topotecan is myelosuppression, consisting mainly of neutropenia. Activity of this semisynthetic analogue of camptothecin has been observed in small cell lung cancer, while its activity in non-small cell lung cancer is not clearly defined, with preliminary data showing low response rates. In ovarian cancer, the activity seems to be modest but definite. The optimal schedule of administration of topotecan has yet to be evaluated by comparing the short-term infusion daily $\times$ 5 q 3–4 weeks with the low-dose 21-day infusion regimen delivered monthly.

More recently, Phase I clinical studies of 9-amino-20(S)-camptothecin (9-AC) have been initiated. There are several i.v. formulations available delivered as a 72-h infusion q 3 weeks or as a continuous infusion escalated by time to 21 days, and later on, by the dose. Based on the experience with 20(S)-camptothecin delivered orally, an oral formulation is being prepared, which may allow a long-term administration. Since 9-AC preclinical data show a wide spectrum of anticancer activity, accelerated clinical studies should be encouraged.

For the two most advanced drugs, CPT-11 and topotecan, there is an urgent need to embark on trials testing combinations with other anticancer drugs. Combination treatments by cisplatin and topo I inhibitors have been initiated in small cell and non-small cell lung cancer in patients with extensive disease. Considering laboratory data, careful attention has to be paid to clinical scheduling of etoposide and other DNA topoisomerase II (topo II) inhibitors combined with camptothecins. In initial studies, topotecan was administered on days 1–3 and etoposide on day 5 or 7–9.[1] In colorectal cancer, combinations will include topo I inhibitors plus 5-Fluorouracil.

One would like further to investigate camptothecins as single agents, using dose escalation and delivery by optimized schedules supported by hemopoietic growth factors. It is obvious that this can be easier for topotecan than CPT-11 should the toxicity profile of the latter be taken into consideration. Besides the combination with hemopoietic growth factors, the concept of dose intensity has to be investigated further, e.g., using the intra-arterial hepatic perfusion by a camptothecin in patients with colon cancer metastases, or an intraperitoneal dwell in patients with advanced cancer of the ovary. Finally, preclinical research of dose-response relationship of camptothecins, and combination additivity or synergism with alkylating agents, should establish whether the drugs can be considered for high-dose chemotherapy with hematopoietic cell support. Dose intensification of CPT-11, however, would most likely result in unpredictable toxicities due to the inherent variability of CPT-11 conversion into its biologically active metabolite SN-38.

It is evident that the studies of DNA topoisomerases, first a laboratory curiosity, opened a new field in chemotherapy. In addition to topo II directed quinolones and related antibiotics used in treatment of infection, and anticancer inhibitors of topo II, camptothecins entered clinical research as a new class of anticancer drugs. Their research may exemplify collaboration between laboratory scientists and clinical researchers, which has been conducted at several institutions in the United States, Japan, and in Europe. The results obtained are encouraging, but unresolved problems remain. Understandably, any more definite evaluation of camptothecin analogues, in terms of their utility in cancer treatments, has to wait until reports of disease-oriented Phase II and randomized trials become available. In conclusion, encouraging Phase I and Phase II trials of CPT-11, and the unprecedented preclinical effectiveness of 9-AC, CAM, and related drugs against major therapy-resistant cancers, warrant intensified clinical research.

REFERENCES

1. The 8th NCI-EORTC symposium on new drugs in cancer therapy, Program and Abstracts, Amsterdam, March 1994.
2. **Niimi, S., Nakagawa, K., Yokota, J., Tsunokawa, Y., Nishio, K., Terashima, Y., Shibuya, M., Terada, M., and Saijo, N.,** Resistance to anticancer drugs in NIH3T3 cells transfected with c-myc and/or c-H-ras gene. *Brit. J. Cancer,* 63: 237–241, 1991.
3. **Mayashita, T. and Reed, J. C.,** Bcl-2 oncoprotein blocks chemotherapy-induced apoptosis in a human leukemia cell line. *Blood,* 81: 151–157, 1993.
4. **Oltval, Z. N., Milliman, C. L., and Korsmeyer, S. J.,** Bcl-2- heterodimerizes *in vivo* with a conserved homolog, bax, that accelerates programmed cell death. *Cell,* 74: 609–619, 1993.
5. **El Rouby, S., Thomas, A., Costin, D., Rosenberg, C. R., Potmesil, M., Silber, R., and Newcomb, E. W.,** p53 gene mutation in B-cell chronic lymphocytic leukemia is associated with drug resistance and is independent of MDR1/MDR3 gene expression. *Blood,* 82: 3452–3459, 1993.
6. **Lowe, S. W., Ruley, H. E., Jacks, T., and Housman, D. E.,** p53 dependent apoptosis modulates the cytotoxicity of anticancer agents. *Cell,* 74: 957–967, 1993.

7. **McGahon, A., Bissonnette, R., Schmitt, M., Cotter, K. M., Green, D. R., and Cotter, T. G.,** BCR-ABL maintains resistance of chronic myelogenous leukemia cells to apoptotic cell death. *Blood,* 83: 1179–1187, 1994.

8. **Hochster, H., Liebes, L., Speyer, J., Sorich, J., Taubes, B., Oratz, J., Wernz, J., Chachoua, A., Raphael, B., Vinci, R. Z., and Blum, R. H.,** Phase I trial of low-dose continuous topotecan infusion in patients with cancer: an active and well-tolerated regimen. *J. Clin. Oncol.,* 12: 553–559, 1994.

INDEX